Neurodiversity in Silence

In a world built for words, *Neurodiversity in Silence* reveals the powerful, often invisible experiences of children and adults living with both Autism Spectrum Disorder (ASD) and hearing impairment. Through the lens of neuroscience, education, and human empathy, Dr. Hina Hadayat Ali and Dr. Hina Fazil invite us to see beyond diagnosis, and into a deeper understanding of minds that communicate differently.

This groundbreaking book uncovers the profound challenges of dual diagnosis: the diagnostic tools that miss the mark, the systems that fail to connect, and the educators left without a map. Yet at its core, *Neurodiversity in Silence* is a story of resilience and reimagining, of children who express through gesture, image, and sensation, and of caregivers and professionals who build bridges across silence. From brain development and sensory processing to multimodal communication and inclusive classrooms, this book equips readers with evidence-based insights and actionable strategies.

Whether you are a teacher, clinician, parent, policymaker, or advocate, you will find guidance, and hope, within these pages. This may also be of interest to students and researchers in special education, psychology, neuroscience, and disability studies.

Hina Hadayat Ali is an Assistant Professor at the University of Education, Lahore (Faisalabad Campus), specializing in neurodevelopmental and sensory impairments, with a focus on autism spectrum disorder. Her research investigates intellectual, sensory, psychological, and neurological factors influencing behaviour, health, and academic achievement, with expertise in applied behaviour analysis, evidence-based interventions, and assistive technology. She advances inclusive education, social integration, and quality of life for individuals with disabilities through research-driven practice.

Hina Fazil is a distinguished academician and researcher with over twenty-five years of experience in intellectual and developmental disabilities, autism, and inclusive education. She serves as an Associate Professor at the Institute of Special Education, University of the Punjab, Lahore, contributing through research, teaching, and supervision of PhD, MPhil, Master's, and BS students, and actively supporting government and NGO initiatives in policy, capacity building, and school reforms. A renowned researcher and author of nine influential books, she has published research articles in top-rated journals and represented Pakistan internationally, establishing herself as a leading figure in special education.

Neurodiversity in Silence

Understanding Dual Diagnosis in Autism and Hearing Impairment

Hina Hadayat Ali and Hina Fazil

Routledge
Taylor & Francis Group
LONDON AND NEW YORK

Designed cover image: Getty Images

First published 2026
by Routledge
4 Park Square, Milton Park, Abingdon, Oxon OX14 4RN

and by Routledge
605 Third Avenue, New York, NY 10158

Routledge is an imprint of the Taylor & Francis Group, an informa business

For Product Safety Concerns and Information please contact our EU representative GPSR@taylorandfrancis.com. Taylor & Francis Verlag GmbH, Kaufingerstraße 24, 80331 München, Germany.

British Library Cataloguing in Publication Data
A catalogue record for this book is available from the British Library

Library of Congress Cataloging-in-Publication Data
A catalog record has been requested for this book

ISBN: 978-1-041-26506-1 (hbk)
ISBN: 978-1-041-26504-7 (pbk)
ISBN: 978-1-003-75061-1 (ebk)

DOI: 10.4324/9781003750611

Typeset in Sabon
by Taylor & Francis Books

Contents

List of tables vi
Acknowledgements x
About the Authors xi
Preface xiii
List of Abbreviations xv

1 Dual Diagnosis Demystified: Autism and Hearing Impairment 1

2 Neurobiological and Sensory Foundations of Co-occurring ASD and Hearing Loss 10

3 Assessment and Diagnostic Challenges in Dual Diagnosis 27

4 Communication and Language Development Across Modalities 43

5 Educational and Behavioral Interventions 66

6 Social-Emotional and Cognitive Development 87

7 Inclusive Policy and Legal Frameworks 105

8 Transition Planning and Lifespan Support 132

Index 154

Tables

1.1 Summary of key aspects of Autism Spectrum Disorder (ASD) 2
1.2 Summary of key aspects of Hearing Impairment 3
1.3 Overview of key components related to Autism Spectrum Disorder and Hearing Impairment 4
1.4 Comparison of key aspects of Autism Spectrum Disorder, Hearing Impairment, and Dual Diagnosis 6
1.5 Major barriers in assessing dual diagnosis of ASD and Hearing Impairment 7
2.1 The comparison highlights key shared and distinct neural mechanisms of Autism Spectrum Disorder and hearing loss, offering insights for accurate diagnosis and effective intervention 12
2.2 A comparative view of auditory processing and sensory integration across ASD, Hearing Impairment, and dual diagnosis to guide accurate understanding and tailored intervention 14
2.3 A comparative overview of genetic, prenatal, and environmental factors influencing ASD, Hearing Impairment, and their overlapping risks to support early identification and integrated intervention 17
2.4 A brief comparison of shared and distinct neural pathways underlying ASD and Hearing Impairment to support clearer neurodevelopmental understanding 21
2.5 A brief comparison of genetic, environmental, and prenatal influences contributing to ASD, Hearing Impairment, and their overlapping developmental risks 23
3.1 Purpose of each tool and adaptations made for Deaf and Hard of Hearing (DHH) children 37
3.2 Primary roles of professionals, including Audiologist, Psychologist, SLP, and Special Educator, in assessment and intervention 39

4.1 Definition, benefits, cognitive, social-emotional, motor, environmental, and educational implications of sign language for children with ASD and Hearing Impairment, including recommended adaptations and overall impact 45
4.2 Key aspects and impacts of sign language for children with ASD and Hearing Impairment, including definition, benefits, cognitive, social-emotional, motor, environmental, educational implications, and adaptations 48
4.3 Challenges in conversational skills, nonverbal communication, social reciprocity, figurative language, perspective-taking, symbolic language, prosody, and exposure to language models for children with ASD, Hearing Impairment, and their combined impact in dual diagnosis, along with recommended support strategies 51
4.4 key bilingual language-support strategies designed to strengthen communication development for children with Hearing Impairment 59
4.5 Accessibility and input modes of speech, sign language, and AAC to guide effective multimodal communication planning 60
4.6 Key factors that significantly shape language and developmental outcomes in children with Hearing Impairment 62
5.1 Essential classroom modifications that support accessibility, communication, sensory needs, instruction, and collaboration for learners with diverse abilities 75
5.2 Key intervention approaches, their primary focus areas, and simple practical examples used with learners 81
5.3 Strategies strengthening home–school collaboration through training, communication, and shared planning 82
6.1 Autism Spectrum Disorder and Hearing Impairment individually affect executive functions, and how their combined presence leads to compounded cognitive and behavioral challenges 95
6.2 Strategies that support mental health, self-advocacy, and social participation by reducing anxiety, building understanding, and strengthening real-life social responses 101
7.1 A unified legal mandate, ensuring inclusive education, accessibility, and individualized support, protecting the rights and needs of learners with dual diagnoses such as ASD and Hearing Impairment 106
7.2 Provisions ensuring individualized, accessible, and family centered support that promotes communication, learning, and inclusion for students with ASD and/or Hearing Impairment 107

7.3 UNCRPD provisions ensuring inclusive education, accessible communication, and supportive learning environments for children with ASD and/or Hearing Impairment through tailored communication tools, accessible classrooms, and active participation in decision-making 109
7.4 Entitlements ensuring equitable, accessible, and individualized education, communication, and support services for children with dual diagnoses, promoting inclusion, development, and family empowerment 110
7.5 Language rights ensuring accessible communication, early exposure, culturally aligned supports, and empowered self-expression for individuals with dual diagnoses, preventing language deprivation and promoting full participation 114
7.6 Challenges highlighting systemic gaps, awareness, resources, enforcement, and coordination that prevent individuals with dual diagnoses from fully accessing their legal rights and essential supports 119
7.7 Barriers reflecting societal stigma, low expectations, and weak community engagement that limit awareness, acceptance, and sustained support for children with dual diagnoses, hindering their inclusion and development 120
7.8 Roles strengthening rights, services, awareness, and accountability, ensuring coordinated advocacy and support for individuals with dual diagnoses across policy, legal, educational, and community systems 122
7.9 The need for early multimodal language access, culturally aligned supports, stronger policies, trained personnel, and inclusive communication systems to address the complex needs of children with dual diagnoses 125
7.10 Policies collectively ensuring inclusive education, accessible environments, and strengthened rights for individuals with dual diagnoses across national and global frameworks 127
7.11 Organizations support health monitoring, awareness, research, accessibility, and cultural representation for individuals with dual diagnoses 128
8.1 Effective transition for individuals with dual diagnoses requiring coordinated planning, accessible education and employment opportunities, self-advocacy support, interagency collaboration, and culturally responsive family and community involvement 135
8.2 Addressing barriers to transition for individuals with dual diagnoses that require inclusive vocational programs, accessible communication, employer awareness, high expectations, coordinated services, mentorship, and supportive social environments 137

8.3 Vocational models emphasizing individualized, strength-based employment and life-skills training with accessible communication, real-world experience, and supportive environments to enhance independence and inclusion for individuals with dual diagnoses 138
8.4 Inclusive post-secondary education for dual-diagnosed students requiring accessible communication, neurodiverse-informed instruction, sensory supports, trained disability services, flexible learning, peer mentoring, and a culturally affirming campus environment 140
8.5 Across life stages, goals progress from school adaptation in early childhood, to self-advocacy in adolescence, and vocational and social independence in adulthood for individuals with dual diagnoses 149
8.6 Supports fostering employment readiness, community participation, and guided decision-making for individuals with dual diagnoses 151

Acknowledgements

To the children who perceive the world through silence and sensation, and to the educators who meet them there with empathy, ingenuity, and unwavering dedication. Your resilience shapes understanding, and your courage gives voice to the unheard. This work is inspired by you.

About the Authors

Dr. Hina Hadayat Ali is an Assistant Professor of Special Education. Her research is focused on sensory, physical, and mental impairments that substantially limit one or more major life activities, and investigating psychological and neurological effects associated with behaviors causing poor health and low academic achievements. Her academic training and research experience have provided her with an excellent background in various disciplines, including: intellectual disability and treatment, developmental disabilities and treatment; Autism Spectrum Disorder and intervention strategies; behavior analyst and behavior management techniques; hearing impairment; visual impairment; physically handicapped segments of population; and genetics epigenetics. She has a broad background in Special Education, with specific training and expertise in experimental and survey researches and secondary data analysis on the biological and psychological overwhelming of inherent pathology of disabilities and disorders, along with integration of persons with disabilities into society to a decent extent of living, and on development and endorsement of national service delivery mechanism for provision of assistive technology for children with autism spectrum disorder, plus empowering persons with disabilities to reduce poverty, empowering students with unique needs to transit in society to lift economy, and on modulating the health of disabled women to lift rural areas. She laid the groundwork by developing effective measures of psychosocial factors, and measures of determining genetic and epigenetic modifiers to adapt and determining healthy mechanisms to modulate the low risks relevant to disabilities and disorders, plus establishing strong ties with community providers that will make it possible to recruit and track participants over time as documented in the publications. In addition, she successfully examined and administered social validity tools developed by triad perceptions with triad methodical levels of the behavioral intervention program. In summary, she has the expertise of leadership, administration, and motivation necessary to successfully carry out the research endeavors. Her long-term research goals involve developing a comprehensive understanding and practice of key developmental pathways and how alterations in gene expression and environmental factors contribute to social stress, poverty, and childhood hardships of persons with disabilities and disorders.

Dr. Hina Fazil, PhD in Special Education, is a distinguished academician and researcher with extensive experience in special education, particularly in the fields of intellectual and developmental disabilities, autism, and inclusive education. Currently serving as an Associate Professor at the Institute of Special Education, University of the Punjab, she has made significant contributions to the field through her research, teaching, and supervision of students, and has credible experience with 25 years in the field. With her keen interest in intellectual and developmental disabilities, autism, and inclusive education, she is engaged with the Government of Punjab, Pakistan, for special educationist capacity building and school reforms. She has a strong liaison with both the Federal and Provincial Government of Pakistan NGOs and INGOs. Moreover, she has worked as a member of task force to formulate National Special education policy. As a renowned researcher, a special educationist, and dedicated professional, she has published more than 108 research papers in highly rated journals, national and international, categorized by HEC in W, X, and Y. She holds the honour of representing Pakistan across many developed countries, including the UK, USA, Australia, and Norway. In her own capacity she has completed nine research projects and is a well-known research scientist with special expertise in conducting survey and experimental research in social sciences. She has contributed magnanimously to both research and academia. She has produced nine highly rated books that are considered best sellers in the field. She has also supervised 12 and completed 9 PhD theses, around 60 MPhils, 290 Master's and 26 BS theses. Her passion for the field and dedication are enormous, inspiring her students to expect even more from her guidance and mentorship.

Preface

The convergence of Autism Spectrum Disorder (ASD) and hearing impairment represents a largely uncharted and often misunderstood domain within the fields of neurodevelopment, education, and communication sciences. While both conditions independently pose significant challenges to development, learning, and inclusion, their co-occurrence, a dual diagnosis, amplifies complexities that traditional models of diagnosis, support, and intervention are often ill-equipped to address. This book, *Neurodiversity in Silence: Understanding Dual Diagnosis in Autism and hearing impairment*, emerges from the urgent need to bridge this gap.

Children and adults with dual diagnoses live at the margins of multiple systems. They are frequently underserved by autism services that lack understanding of Deaf culture and audiological needs, and by hearing loss support systems that may not account for the social, behavioral, and cognitive nuances of autism. Diagnostic overshadowing, communication barriers, and lack of culturally and linguistically responsive tools contribute to under-identification, misdiagnosis, and fragmented service delivery. Educators, therapists, families, and policymakers are often left without a cohesive framework to support these individuals. This book is an effort to change that.

Neurodiversity in Silence: Understanding Dual Diagnosis in Autism and hearing impairment adopts a holistic, interdisciplinary, and neurodiversity-affirming approach. It begins by laying a foundational understanding of ASD and hearing impairment as distinct yet overlapping conditions, both biologically and behaviorally. It further explores how dual diagnosis affects brain development, sensory integration, language acquisition, and social communication, domains that are critical to human connection and learning (Clark & Adams, 2023).

One of the central tenets of this work is that communication is not confined to speech and that silence is not a void but a different modality of expression. The book emphasizes visual language strategies, multimodal communication supports, and the necessity of accessible environments that recognize the diversity of human minds and bodies. Grounded in current research yet deeply connected to practice, it offers assessment guidelines, intervention strategies, and educational models that honor the unique profiles of individuals with dual diagnoses (Cekaite & Ekström, 2022).

This text was written for a diverse audience, educators, clinicians, researchers, families, and students, who seek to understand, support, and advocate for individuals who live at the intersection of silence and spectrum. It is meant to challenge deficit-based paradigms and replace them with frameworks of possibility, resilience, and respect. It insists that children with ASD and hearing impairment are not puzzles to be solved but people to be understood, each with their own rhythm, language, and way of being in the world.

The chapters that follow are grounded in both scientific evidence and human experience. They invite readers to engage not only intellectually but empathetically, to rethink traditional boundaries between diagnosis and identity, and to co-create systems of care that are inclusive by design.

In compiling this work, we are deeply grateful to the families, educators, researchers, and professionals who contribute daily to the lives of those with dual diagnoses; your insights and advocacy are woven throughout this book. To the children and adults who live Neurodiversity in Silence: Understanding Dual Diagnosis in Autism and hearing impairment, this book is for you, and because of you.

References

Clark, M. L., & Adams, R. D. (2023). Behavioral and social interventions for children with autism: Evidence-based classroom strategies. *Journal of Autism and Developmental Practice*, 12(3), 145–160.

Cekaite, A., & Ekström, A. (2022). Inclusive teaching practices for diverse learners: Multimodal communication and classroom strategies. *Education Inquiry*, *13(1)*, 45–62. doi:10.1080/20004508.2022.2056789.

List of Abbreviations

Acronym	Description
AAC	Augmentative and Alternative Communication
ABA	Applied Behavior Analysis
ABR	Auditory Brainstem Response
ADA	Americans with Disabilities Act
ADI-R	Autism Diagnostic Interview – Revised
ADOS	Autism Diagnostic Observation Schedule
ASD	Autism Spectrum Disorder
ASSQ-DC	Autism Spectrum Screening Questionnaire – Deaf Children
ASL	American Sign Language
BSL	British Sign Language
CDC	Centers for Disease Control and Prevention
CARS	Childhood Autism Rating Scale
CMV	Cytomegalovirus
DHH	Deaf or Hard of Hearing
DSP	Developmental Social-Pragmatic
DTT	Discrete Trial Training
FCT	Functional Communication Training
FM System	Frequency Modulation System
GJB2	Gap Junction Beta-2 (a gene linked to hearing loss)
IDEA	Individuals with Disabilities Education Act
IEP	Individualized Education Program
IFSP	Individualized Family Service Plan
MDT	Multidisciplinary Team

M-CHAT-R	Modified Checklist for Autism in Toddlers – Revised
NICU	Neonatal Intensive Care Unit
OAE	Otoacoustic Emissions
OT	Occupational Therapy / Therapist
PECS	Picture Exchange Communication System
PSL	Pakistan Sign Language
PRT	Pivotal Response Treatment
SGD	Speech-Generating Device
SCQ-DA	Social Communication Questionnaire – Deaf Adaptation
SHANK3, MECP2, CHD8, NRXN1	Genes commonly associated with ASD
SLP	Speech-Language Pathologist
TEACCH	Treatment and Education of Autistic and Communication-Handicapped Children
UDL	Universal Design for Learning
UNCRPD	United Nations Convention on the Rights of Persons with Disabilities
VABS	Vineland Adaptive Behavior Scales

Chapter 1

Dual Diagnosis Demystified

Autism and Hearing Impairment

Overview of Autism Spectrum Disorder (ASD) and hearing impairment

Autism Spectrum Disorder (ASD) and hearing impairment are two distinct neurodevelopmental and sensory conditions that significantly influence an individual's communication, social interaction, and learning processes. When these conditions co-occur, a phenomenon often referred to as dual diagnosis, they present a complex profile of strengths and challenges that require specialized understanding, assessment, and intervention strategies (Centers for Disease Control and Prevention (CDC), 2023).

Autism Spectrum Disorder (ASD)

Autism spectrum disorder (ASD) is characterized by persistent deficits in social communication and interaction, alongside restricted, repetitive patterns of behavior, interests, or activities. The manifestation of these characteristics varies widely in severity, hence the term "spectrum." Individuals with ASD may struggle with understanding social cues, developing peer relationships, using and interpreting verbal and nonverbal communication, and adapting to changes in routines or environments. ASD affects approximately 1 in 36 children in the United States, with prevalence rates rising globally due to increased awareness and improved diagnostic practices (American Psychiatric Association, 2013).

Hearing Impairment

Hearing Impairment (HI), on the other hand, refers to partial or complete inability to hear. It ranges from mild hearing loss to profound deafness and can be congenital or acquired. Depending on the degree and type, conductive, sensorineural, or mixed, hearing loss can impact language development, academic achievement, and social participation. Individuals who are deaf or hard of hearing (DHH) may rely on various communication modes, including

DOI: 10.4324/9781003750611-1

Table 1.1. Summary of key aspects of Autism Spectrum Disorder (ASD)

Aspect	*Details*
Definition	A neurodevelopmental disorder marked by persistent deficits in social communication and interaction, and restricted, repetitive behaviors.
Core Characteristics	Difficulty with social-emotional reciprocity. Challenges in nonverbal communication. Struggles in developing and maintaining relationships.
Behavioral Patterns	Repetitive movements or speech. Insistence on sameness. Intense interests. Sensory sensitivities.
Spectrum Nature	Wide variability in abilities, language use, cognitive functioning, and independence levels.
Communication Challenges	Delayed or absent speech. Limited understanding of social cues. Literal interpretation of language.
Prevalence	Affects 1 in 36 children in the U.S.A. (CDC, 2023); rates increasing globally due to greater awareness and improved diagnostics.
Diagnosis Age Range	Typically identified between 2–4 years old, but may be diagnosed earlier or later depending on symptom presentation.
Gender Ratio	More common in boys than girls (approximately 4:1), though girls may be underdiagnosed due to different symptom profiles.
Causes and Risk Factors	Complex interplay of genetic and environmental factors; no single known cause.

spoken language (with or without assistive devices), sign language, or a combination of both (Davidson & Quittner, 2020).

When ASD and hearing impairment co-occur, their overlapping and contrasting features can complicate diagnosis and intervention. For instance, language delays in children with hearing loss may be mistakenly attributed to autism, and vice versa. Similarly, limited eye contact, social withdrawal, or repetitive behaviors seen in children with hearing impairment may mimic ASD symptoms. This overlap often leads to underdiagnosis or misdiagnosis, especially in young children, ultimately delaying early intervention, which is critical for optimal outcomes.

From a clinical and educational standpoint, individuals with dual diagnosis face unique challenges that extend beyond the sum of their individual conditions. Communication barriers are particularly pronounced; children may have limited access to both auditory input and social-pragmatic learning

Table 1.2. Summary of key aspects of Hearing Impairment

Aspect	*Details*
Definition	Partial or complete inability to hear; can affect one or both ears.
Range of Severity	Mild. Difficulty hearing soft sounds. Moderate. Difficulty understanding speech. Severe to Profound. Little to no hearing.
Types of Hearing Loss	Conductive. Outer or middle ear issues. Sensorineural. Inner ear or auditory nerve damage. Mixed. Combination of both.
Onset	Congenital. Present at birth. Acquired. Occurs later due to illness, injury, noise exposure, or aging.
Impact Areas	Language development. May delay speech and language skills. Academic achievement. Can affect learning and literacy Social participation. May hinder peer interactions and emotional development.
Communication Modes	Spoken language (with/without hearing aids or cochlear implants). Sign language (e.g., ASL, BSL). Total communication (combined modes).
Assistive Technologies	Hearing aids. Cochlear implants. FM systems. Captioning and alerting devices.
Educational Support Needs	Speech therapy. Special education services. Classroom accommodations. Access to interpreters.
Terminology	Deaf. Profound hearing loss, often identifies with deaf culture. Hard of Hearing (HoH). Partial hearing, may use spoken language.

Table 1.3. Overview of key components related to Autism Spectrum Disorder and Hearing Impairment

Component	*Description*
Title	Overview of Autism Spectrum Disorder and Hearing Impairment
Nature of Conditions	ASD and Hearing Impairment are distinct neurodevelopmental and sensory conditions.
Impact Areas	These conditions influence communication, social interaction, and learning processes.
Dual Diagnosis	When ASD and Hearing Impairment co-occur, it is referred to as a dual diagnosis. This combination requires specialized understanding, assessment, and intervention.
Autism Spectrum Disorder (ASD)	Characterized by persistent deficits in social communication and interaction. Individuals exhibit restricted, repetitive patterns of behavior, interests, or activities.
Variability	Manifestations of ASD vary in severity, forming a broad "spectrum."
Common Challenges in ASD	Difficulties with social cues, peer relationships, verbal and nonverbal communication, and adapting to change.
Prevalence	Affects approximately 1 in 36 children in the U.S.A.; global rates are increasing due to awareness and better diagnosis.

opportunities, affecting their expressive and receptive language development (Davidson & Quittner, 2020). Sensory sensitivities common in ASD may be exacerbated by the need for hearing aids or cochlear implants, and vice versa. Social isolation, behavioral issues, and academic difficulties are also more prevalent in this population.

Factors Contributing to Under Identification

Several factors contribute to this under-identification, as follows:

Symptom Overlap

Both ASD and hearing impairment can present with limited speech, poor eye contact, and difficulties with social interaction. Without appropriate assessment tools and interdisciplinary expertise, it becomes difficult to differentiate whether these behaviors are due to auditory deprivation or neurodevelopmental differences (Hall & Samar, 2020).

Inadequate Training Among Professionals

Many audiologists, speech-language pathologists, psychologists, and educators may not be sufficiently trained to recognize dual diagnoses. A professional with expertise in hearing loss may lack familiarity with autism traits and vice versa, leading to incomplete assessments.

Lack of Culturally and Linguistically Appropriate Tools

Standard diagnostic instruments such as the Autism Diagnostic Observation Schedule (ADOS) or the Childhood Autism Rating Scale (CARS) are designed for verbal, typically hearing children and may not yield valid results when applied to DHH children. This can lead to false negatives or inconclusive findings.

Communication Barriers in Assessment

When a child uses sign language or an alternative communication mode, and the evaluator lacks proficiency in those modes, important behaviors or social nuances may be misinterpreted, again contributing to missed or incorrect diagnoses.

Parental and Societal Perceptions

1 In many cases, families may resist or question the possibility of a second diagnosis due to stigma, fear, or lack of awareness.
2 Cultural norms and limited access to specialized diagnostic services in low-resource settings further compound the issue.
3 Addressing diagnostic overshadowing and under-identification requires a paradigm shift toward interdisciplinary, bias-aware, and disability-affirmative diagnostic practices.
4 Assessment teams must include professionals with dual expertise in ASD and hearing impairment and employ adapted, validated tools that consider both auditory and neurodevelopmental contexts.
5 Equally important is the incorporation of parent insights, communication mode assessments, and observations across naturalistic settings.

Hence, the interplay of diagnostic overshadowing and under-identification poses a significant barrier to timely and accurate diagnosis of co-occurring ASD and hearing impairment. Raising awareness among professionals, developing inclusive assessment protocols, and strengthening interdisciplinary collaboration are critical to ensuring that all children receive the support and services they need to thrive.

The comparative paradigm outlines the differentiating and intersecting features of ASD, and the hearing impairment (HI) and their concomitant

Table 1.4. Comparison of key aspects of Autism Spectrum Disorder, Hearing Impairment, and Dual Diagnosis

Aspect	*ASD*	*Hearing Impairment*	*Dual Diagnosis*
Core Features	Social communication challenges, repetitive behaviors.	Limited hearing, speech delay.	Combination of both challenges.
Causes	Neurodevelopmental and genetic factors.	Sensorineural or conductive deficits.	Overlap of both etiologies.
Interventions	Behavioral therapy, communication training.	Hearing aids, speech therapy.	Multimodal support, interdisciplinary approach.

occurrence in a Dual Diagnosis. The triadic comparison is used as an analytic base in interpreting the unique and interactive effect of each condition on development, communication and intervention planning.

ASD is a rather complicated neurodevelopmental disorder, which is marked by a perennial lack of social communication skills and limited or stereotypical behavior. People with ASD tend to have an abnormal social-reciprocity, inability to understand nonverbal communication, and an increase or decrease in sensorial responses. ASD has mainly neurobiological and genetic etiological roots, with the changes occurring in the connections of the brain, as well as the regulation of synaptic activity (De Rubeis and Buxbaum, 2015). Interventions are mostly behavioral and communicative, such as Applied Behavior Analysis (ABA), Social Communication Therapy, and the application of Augmentative and Alternative Communication (AAC) in order to establish better interaction.

hearing impairment (HI) on the other hand is a sensorial disorder caused by the impairments in the auditory perception, and this may be conductive, sensorineural or mixed. It affects it mainly linguistically and socially because when auditory input is reduced, the access to phonological structures, prosody and incidental language learning is limited (Davidson & Quittner, 2020). Etiology is most frequently sensorineural damage, genetic abnormality (e.g. GJB2 mutations – for this and other abbreviations, please see their full form at the beginning of this book), infection, or environmental. Treatment of HI is generally audiological and speech-based, comprising the use of hearing aids, cochlear implants, and speech-language therapy, and sign language and total communication strategies have guaranteed equal access to language.

The Dual Diagnosis, the overlap of the ASD and HI, generates an unfamiliar neurodevelopmental and communicative profile which cannot be properly handled by addressing each condition separately. The person faces a combination of difficulty in sound processing, social cognitions and sensory management, which leads to extreme difficulties in both expressive and receptive communications. The etiological basis is frequently multifactorial with an overlap of neurodevelopmental factors with anomalies of the auditory system. The interventions should thus be multimodal and interdisciplinary integrating the behavioral, audiological, sensory-integration and educational interventions to facilitate the holistic development. Audiologists, psychologists, speech-language pathologists, and special educators should work together in order to maximize results.

This relative insight emphasizes the fact that although both ASD and hearing impairment play different roles in communication, their interactional interplay creates an interactional effect, which has a compounding effect on the development. The dual diagnosis dictates other inclusive assessment practices to consider both the social-communicative and the auditory access, without the overshadowing of the diagnosis. Also, evidence-based multimodal interventions based on neurodiversity-affirming models continue to be at the forefront in ensuring meaningful participation, adaptive functioning as well as quality of life among individuals who experience both silence and spectrum.

The issue of correct diagnosis of co-occurring ASD and hearing impairment (HI) is highly complicated in terms of its diagnosis; see Table 1.2, which shows the key factors that hinder effective evaluation and early treatment. All obstacles, symptom similarity, absence of modified diagnostic measures, and cultural prejudice are systemic issues with clinical and situational constraints.

The most ubiquitous impediment of proper diagnosis involves Symptom Overlap. Most of the fundamental behaviors related to ASD, including the lack of eye contact, speech delays, repetitive behaviors, and social withdrawal, might also occur as coping mechanisms of having auditory deprivation in hearing-impaired children (Hall & Samar, 2020). An example is when a deaf child appears not to be listening or paying attention, or when they seem not to respond to verbal communication, it might occur that he or she is attempting to communicate through hand gestures instead of being stereotypical because of repetitive actions. Unless audiological and developmental assessments are conducted in detail, such behaviors can be wrongly attributed by the professionals, leading to diagnostic overshadowing, a situation where a condition hides or is confused with another one. This interlude also highlights the necessity of multidisciplinary evaluation and the application of behaviorally and linguistically delicate observation models that distinguish between neurodevelopmental and sensory manifestations.

Table 1.5. Major barriers in assessing dual diagnosis of ASD and Hearing Impairment

Barrier	*Description*
Symptom Overlap	Similar behavioral patterns confuse differentiation.
Lack of Tools	Most assessments not adapted for DHH populations.
Cultural Bias	Limited awareness among professionals and families.

Diagnostic uncertainty is further increased by the lack of tools. The majority of standardized testing tools of autism, including the Autism Diagnostic Observation Schedule (ADOS), Autism Diagnostic Interview-Revised (ADI-R), or the Modified Checklist for Autism in Toddlers (M-CHAT-R), were standardized in hearing or verbally fluent groups (Lord et al., 2012). As a result, they do not take into consideration linguistic, sensory and cultural peculiarities of Deaf and Hard of Hearing (DHH) people. The most important communicative subtleties that are conveyed by means of sign language, visual attention, or gesture can be missed or misunderstood by those who do not know sign language. Equity in diagnosis and the timely provision of necessary intervention has not been achieved because there are no validated instruments, such as the Social Communication Questionnaire – Deaf Adaptation (SCQ-DA) or the Autism Spectrum Screening Questionnaire – Deaf Children (ASSQ-DC), used in everyday clinical practice.

Therefore, culturally and linguistically sensitive diagnostic instruments have to be developed and disseminated in order to minimize false positives and negatives in dual-diagnostic groups.

A third and in most cases unidentified barrier is Cultural Bias. The programs of professional training and diagnostic paradigms are mostly based on the hearing-centric and Western clinical models that might not be effective in a variety of diverse linguistic and cultural environments (Deaf Child Worldwide, 2021). There can also be differences in the perceptions of disability between families and practitioners whereby some may believe that deafness as a linguistic identity and not as an impairment whereas others may be reluctant to receive another label like autism because of stigma or fear. Furthermore, inexperienced evaluators that do not understand deaf culture and bilingual-bimodal development might pathologize culturally normative behaviors in the sign-using communities, including emphatic facial expressions or changes in gaze taken to indicate a turn. Such cultural and linguistic disparities continue to maintain misdiagnosis, underdiagnosis, or service omission.

All these impediments highlight the need to have inclusive, bias-sensitive and interdisciplinary diagnostic models. The professionals should be prepared to identify the interaction of sensory and neurodevelopmental factors, use modified assessment instruments, and collaborate with the family and cultural intermediaries to achieve diagnostic validity. Through the systemic changes suggested in Table 1.2, the clinicians and educators will be able to shift towards more equitable methods of identification that would respect the neurological diversity and cultural-linguistic identity of people living with the dual diagnosis.

Real-Life Situation: The Early Detection of Dual Diagnosis

Ayesha was three years old; she showed little speech and was hardly responsive to her name being called. She was first diagnosed with autistic syndrome, and she began attending sign-oriented sessions in an early intervention center. An audiologist who came to check them recommended an auditory screening, which showed severe bilateral hearing loss. As soon as hearing aids were installed and sessions were introduced with a combination of sign language and social-communication therapy, Ayesha became much more engaged. This case demonstrates the necessity of multidisciplinary screening to identify the common characteristics between ASD and hearing impairment, and provide the necessary support in time and in the most effective way.

Summary

1 Autism Spectrum Disorder (ASD) and hearing impairment are similar but different disorders that affect communication, learning, and social interaction.
2 Dual diagnosis exacerbates developmental and behavioral problems, and requires special, interpersonal reactions.
3 Overdiagnosis and misdiagnosis often lead to late intervention.
4 Integrated audiological and behavioral diagnostic practice will be more accurate owing to the inclusive diagnostic practices.
5 Early detection, family education and working together as a professional are proving better results and involvement.

References

American Psychiatric Association. (2013). *Diagnostic and statistical manual of mental disorders* (5th edn.). American Psychiatric Publishing. doi:10.1176/appi.books.9780890425596.

Centers for Disease Control and Prevention (CDC). (2023). *Data and statistics on autism spectrum disorder (ASD)*. U.S. Department of Health & Human Services. https://www.cdc.gov/ncbddd/autism/data.html.

Davidson, L. S., & Quittner, A. L. (2020). Parenting children with hearing loss: Emotional, behavioral, and social development. In M. Marschark & H. Knoors (Eds.), *The Oxford Handbook of Deaf Studies in Learning and Cognition*. Oxford University Press.

De Rubeis, S., & Buxbaum, J. D. (2015). Genetics and genomics of autism spectrum disorder. *Current Neurology and Neuroscience Reports*, 15(7), 1–9. doi:10.1007/s11910-015-0574-4.

Deaf Child Worldwide. (2021). *Barriers to inclusive education for deaf children*. Deaf Child Worldwide. https://www.deafchildworldwide.info.

Hall, W. C., & Samar, V. J. (2020). Impact of hearing loss on social and cognitive development in autistic and non-autistic children. *Journal of Deaf Studies and Deaf Education*, 25(2), 123–135. doi:10.1093/deafed/enz047.

Lord, C., Rutter, M., DiLavore, P., Risi, S., Gotham, K., & Bishop, S. (2012). *Autism Diagnostic Observation Schedule (ADOS-2)* (2nd edn.). Western Psychological Services.

Chapter 2

Neurobiological and Sensory Foundations of Co-occurring ASD and Hearing Loss

Shared and Divergent Neural Pathways in ASD and Hearing Loss

Understanding the neurobiological underpinnings of Autism Spectrum Disorder (ASD) and hearing loss reveals both shared and divergent neural pathways, which can inform diagnostic precision and targeted interventions for individuals with a dual diagnosis.

While ASD and hearing impairment are distinct conditions, one neurodevelopmental and the other sensory, they may intersect at the level of brain development, neural connectivity, and sensory processing, thereby influencing behavior, cognition, and communication.

Shared Neural Pathways and Intersections

Both conditions may be associated with atypical auditory cortex development, though arising from distinct mechanisms related to sensory deprivation in hearing loss and neurodevelopmental differences in ASD.

In children with congenital hearing loss, decreased or absent auditory input results in reduced stimulation to the auditory pathways, leading to structural and functional changes in the brain, including cortical reorganization.

Another point of convergence lies in the mirror neuron system, which is crucial for imitation, empathy, and social interaction. This system is often underactive in individuals with ASD and may also be affected in children with hearing loss due to reduced opportunities for social-linguistic modeling and feedback during early development. This shared disruption contributes to difficulties in joint attention, theory of mind, and social reciprocity in both populations (Anderson & Haegele, 2023).

Moreover, atypical connectivity within and between key brain networks, such as the default mode network (DMN), salience network, and language networks, has been reported in both ASD and children with auditory deprivation (Hall & Samar, 2020). These shared patterns of dysconnectivity may help

DOI: 10.4324/9781003750611-2

explain overlapping behavioral features such as communication difficulties, sensory sensitivities, and social disengagement (Buckner et al., 2008).

Divergent Neural Mechanisms

Despite shared features, the underlying causes and specific neural mechanisms of ASD and hearing loss are fundamentally different. ASD is primarily associated with genetic and neurodevelopmental factors, including mutations in genes regulating synaptic function and neural plasticity (e.g., SHANK3, MECP2, NRXN1). Brain imaging studies in ASD show atypical growth trajectories such as early brain overgrowth, reduced white matter integrity, and aberrant connectivity patterns, particularly in frontal and temporal regions (De Rubeis & Buxbaum, 2015).

In contrast, hearing loss is often linked to peripheral deficits, in the cochlea, auditory nerve, or brainstem pathways. While congenital hearing loss may indirectly affect cortical development due to reduced sensory input, its root cause is usually anatomical, infectious, or genetic (e.g., GJB2 mutations), and it primarily affects auditory transmission and perception rather than broader cognitive and social domains (Smith et al., 2005).

Furthermore, brain plasticity in hearing loss often results in cross-modal reorganization, where regions of the brain typically reserved for auditory processing are repurposed for visual or tactile functions. This phenomenon is less common in ASD, where multisensory integration is often impaired rather than repurposed.

Implications for Dual Diagnosis

There are four main implications for dual diagnosis, as follows:

1. Understanding both the overlapping and unique neural characteristics of ASD and hearing loss is critical for accurate diagnosis and effective intervention.
2. The presence of shared neural vulnerabilities, such as delayed auditory processing or impaired social cognition, may increase the likelihood of co-occurrence, while divergent pathways highlight the importance of distinguishing each condition based on etiology and neurodevelopmental profile.
3. Intervention strategies must reflect this complexity. For example, children with ASD and hearing loss may benefit from approaches that combine auditory habilitation (e.g., cochlear implants, hearing aids) with autism-specific therapies targeting social communication, sensory regulation, and executive functioning.
4. Additionally, neuroimaging research may lead to **biomarkers** that can assist in early identification and personalized treatment planning for individuals with dual diagnoses.

Table 2.1. The comparison highlights key shared and distinct neural mechanisms of Autism Spectrum Disorder and hearing loss, offering insights for accurate diagnosis and effective intervention

Aspect	*Description*
Purpose	To understand shared and divergent neural mechanisms underlying ASD and hearing loss, aiding diagnostic accuracy and intervention design.
Nature of Conditions	ASD: Neurodevelopmental disorder. Hearing Loss: Sensory impairment. Both impact brain development and sensory processing.
Shared Neural Pathways	**Description**
Auditory Cortex Development	Atypical development noted in both conditions; in hearing loss, due to lack of auditory input; in ASD, due to neurodevelopmental anomalies.
Cortical Reorganization	Found in congenital hearing loss due to sensory deprivation. May influence brain regions overlapping with ASD-related deficits.
Mirror Neuron System	Underactive in ASD; also affected in hearing loss due to reduced social-linguistic exposure, impacting social-emotional development and joint attention.
Brain Network Dysconnectivity	Atypical connectivity in DMN, salience, and language networks in both ASD and auditory deprivation, contributing to shared symptoms (e.g., communication deficits, sensory sensitivities).
Divergent Neural Mechanisms	**Description**
Etiology	ASD: Genetic mutations (e.g., SHANK3, MECP2, NRXN1). Hearing Loss: Peripheral anatomical, infectious, or genetic causes (e.g., GJB2 mutations).
Brain Structure and Function	ASD: Abnormal brain growth, reduced white matter, aberrant frontal/temporal connectivity. Hearing Loss: Affects auditory nerve, cochlea, brainstem.
Sensory Reorganization	Hearing Loss: Cross-modal plasticity (auditory areas used for vision/touch). ASD: Impaired multisensory integration, not typically repurposed.

Auditory Processing and Sensory Integration Differences

Auditory processing and sensory integration are critical components of human development, shaping how individuals perceive, interpret, and respond to their environment.

Auditory Processing in ASD and hearing impairment

Auditory processing refers to how the brain interprets and makes sense of sound input. In individuals with hearing impairment, auditory processing deficits are primarily the result of diminished or distorted auditory input due to damage or dysfunction in the outer, middle, or inner ear, or along the auditory nerve (Baron-Cohen et al., 2013).

When ASD and hearing impairment co-occur, the clinical picture becomes more complex. A child may have reduced access to sound due to hearing loss and simultaneously experience auditory hypersensitivity due to autism-related sensory processing issues. These dual challenges can obscure the origin of observed behaviors and necessitate highly individualized auditory and sensory evaluations.

Sensory Integration Differences

Sensory integration is the neurological process that organizes sensory input from the body and environment to enable effective interaction with the world. Both ASD and hearing impairment are associated with distinct patterns of sensory integration difficulties.

In ASD, sensory processing differences are recognized as core features of the disorder. The DSM-5 includes hyper- or hyporeactivity to sensory input and unusual interest in sensory aspects of the environment as diagnostic criteria. Many individuals with ASD experience difficulties integrating information across multiple sensory modalities (e.g., sound, touch, vision), which can affect attention, motor coordination, and emotional regulation. For instance, a child may become overwhelmed by background noise while trying to interpret facial expressions, resulting in withdrawal or behavioral outbursts.

For individuals with hearing impairment, sensory integration challenges may arise as a compensatory response to limited auditory input. Enhanced reliance on visual, tactile, and proprioceptive input is common. Cross-modal plasticity, whereby brain areas traditionally dedicated to hearing are reorganized to process visual or somatosensory information, can enhance visual attention and spatial awareness (Kral & Sharma, 2012). However, this reorganization may also contribute to altered sensory experiences and require specific support in balancing sensory inputs, especially in multisensory learning environments.

Table 2.2. **A comparative view of auditory processing and sensory integration across ASD, Hearing Impairment, and dual diagnosis to guide accurate understanding and tailored intervention**

Domain	*Autism Spectrum Disorder*	*Hearing Impairment*	*Dual Diagnosis (ASD + HI)*
Auditory Processing	Auditory hypersensitivity or hyposensitivity. Delayed or distorted interpretation of sounds.	Reduced or distorted input due to damage in ear structures or auditory nerve.	Combined auditory deprivation and sensory overload. Difficulty localizing sound sources or filtering background noise.
Behavioral Manifestations	Avoidance of loud environments. Overreaction to normal sounds. Sound-seeking behaviors.	Difficulty detecting or distinguishing speech sounds. Delays in speech/language.	Confusing behavioral cues (e.g., is a child ignoring due to sensory overload or lack of hearing?).
Sensory Integration	Core feature of ASD Hyper/hyporesponsiveness to sensory input. Difficulty integrating multisensory information.	Compensatory reliance on visual/tactile/proprioceptive input. Altered body awareness.	Complex sensory profile. May rely heavily on visual cues while struggling with simultaneous stimuli.
Neurological Basis	Atypical connectivity in sensory brain regions. Overactivation or underactivation of sensory cortices.	Cross-modal plasticity (auditory cortex re-purposed). Enhanced visual processing.	Brain may be under dual adaptation stress. Need for customized neurodevelopmental assessments.
Learning Implications	Challenges in attention, emotional regulation, and social interaction. May benefit from sensory diets.	May need visual/kinesthetic support. Delayed academic skills.	High need for multisensory-balanced learning. Potential misinterpretation of behaviors by educators.
Assessment Needs	Sensory profile assessments. Auditory filtering and attention tests.	Audiological exams. Functional hearing and speech perception tests.	Integrated, interdisciplinary evaluations. Consider both hearing loss and sensory integration issues.

Domain	*Autism Spectrum Disorder*	*Hearing Impairment*	*Dual Diagnosis (ASD + HI)*
Support Strategies	Sensory-friendly environments. Structured routines and visual supports.	Use of hearing aids or cochlear implants. Sign language or total communication.	Individualized sensory and communication plans. Avoid over-stimulation while maximizing accessible input.

Educational and Therapeutic Implications

Listed here are four of the educational and therapeutic implications.

1 It is essential to understand auditory and sensory processing profiles is essential for designing effective interventions.
2 Integrated sensory assessments by occupational therapssts, audiologists, and behavior specialists can help identify individual sensory patterns. Interventions such as sensory integration therapy, auditory-verbal therapy, or structured teaching with visual supports can be tailored to reduce sensory overload and enhance functional communication.
3 Educators and therapists must create sensory-friendly learning environments, minimizing unpredictable noise, providing clear visual schedules, using tactile supports, and allowing sensory breaks.
4 In dual-diagnosis populations, the combination of hearing technology (e.g., cochlear implants or hearing aids) with sensory-based strategies can promote better regulation, engagement, and learning outcomes (Soorya & Tang, 2022).

Role of genetics, environmental risks, and prenatal factors

The co-occurrence of Autism Spectrum Disorder (ASD) and hearing impairment is a multifactorial phenomenon influenced by a complex interplay of genetic predispositions, environmental exposures, and prenatal factors. Understanding these contributing elements not only enhances our insight into the etiology of dual diagnoses but also supports the development of targeted screening, preventive strategies, and early interventions.

Genetic Contributions

Both ASD and hearing loss have strong genetic components. ASD is associated with numerous genetic variants, including rare de novo mutations and common polygenic risk factors. Some well-documented genetic syndromes, such as Fragile X Syndrome, Rett Syndrome, and Tuberous Sclerosis, present with autistic features and may also include auditory processing abnormalities or hearing issues. Research has identified mutations in genes involved in synaptic function, neural connectivity, and brain development (e.g., SHANK3, MECP2, CHD8) as contributing to ASD phenotypes (Hagerman & Hagerman, 2002).

Hearing impairment, particularly congenital forms, is also frequently genetic in origin. More than 50% of prelingual hearing loss in developed countries is attributed to genetic causes, with mutations in genes such as GJB2, GJB6, and SLC26A4 being common culprits. These genes affect the structure and function of the inner ear and auditory pathways.

In some cases, shared genetic mechanisms may contribute to the dual presentation of ASD and hearing loss. For example, mitochondrial disorders or chromosomal abnormalities (e.g., deletions on chromosome 15q or 22q) can affect multiple systems, including both neural development and auditory function. Additionally, some forms of syndromic deafness (e.g., Usher Syndrome, Waardenburg Syndrome) may include cognitive, behavioral, or social communication features similar to those seen in ASD.

Environmental Risk Factors

Here are four environmental risk factors that should be considered.

1. Beyond genetics, various environmental exposures have been implicated in the etiology of both ASD and hearing loss. These may include prenatal infections (e.g., rubella, cytomegalovirus, or toxoplasmosis), maternal substance use, toxic exposures (e.g., heavy metals like mercury or lead), and perinatal complications (e.g., hypoxia, low birth weight, prematurity).
2. Cytomegalovirus (CMV) infection during pregnancy is a notable example, as it is a leading cause of non-genetic congenital hearing loss and has also been linked to increased autism risk in some studies (Lanzieri et al., 2014).
3. Similarly, maternal exposure to valproic acid, an antiepileptic drug, has been associated with a higher likelihood of both ASD and sensorineural hearing impairment in offspring. These findings emphasize the role of teratogenic agents and their effects on fetal brain and sensory organ development (Christensen et al., 2013).
4. Environmental stressors, such as poor prenatal care, malnutrition, or exposure to high-stress environments, may exacerbate genetic vulnerabilities, triggering atypical neural development through epigenetic mechanisms (Burke & Hodapp, 2020). These factors may not directly cause either condition but can modulate gene expression in ways that increase susceptibility (Brookman-Frazee et al., 2006).

Table 2.3. **A comparative overview of genetic, prenatal, and environmental factors influencing ASD, Hearing Impairment, and their overlapping risks to support early identification and integrated intervention**

Factor Category	*Autism Spectrum Disorder*	*Hearing Impairment*	*Shared/Overlapping Risk for Dual Diagnosis*
Genetic Basis	Involves rare de novo mutations and common polygenic variants. Key genes: SHANK3, CHD8, MECP2.	Over 50% of congenital hearing loss is genetic. Common genes: GJB2, GJB6, SLC26A4.	Some genetic syndromes (e.g., Rett, Fragile X, Tuberous Sclerosis) show both ASD traits and hearing loss.
Syndromic Links	Found in syndromes with multiple developmental anomalies.	Present in syndromic deafness (e.g., Usher, Waardenburg).	Shared syndromes often affect neural and auditory development (e.g., 22q11 deletion, mitochondrial disorders).
Chromosomal Abnormalities	Deletions or duplications in regions like 15q11–13, 16p11.2, 22q13.	May involve chromosomal abnormalities affecting inner ear development.	Overlapping chromosomal deletions (e.g., 22q, 15q) linked to both auditory and neurodevelopmental impairments.
Prenatal Risk Factors	Maternal infections (e.g., rubella, CMV). Advanced parental age. Prenatal exposure to toxins (e.g., valproate).	Intrauterine infections (e.g., CMV, rubella). Hypoxia or prematurity. Ototoxic drug exposure.	Shared prenatal insults can disrupt brain and ear development (e.g., CMV, rubella, hypoxia).
Environmental Influences	Early life stressors. Environmental toxins. Perinatal complications.	Noise trauma. Meningitis. NICU stays with ototoxic medications.	Shared exposure to environmental risks may amplify vulnerability in genetically predisposed individuals.
Implications for Screening	Need for genetic counseling and early neurodevelopmental screening.	Universal newborn hearing screening and genetic testing for etiology.	Integrated early screening protocols recommended for high-risk infants or those with atypical sensory/social development.
Preventive/Early Action	Early intervention services. Parent education. Genetic testing if syndromic signs present.	Use of hearing aids/ cochlear implants. Early speech/ language therapy.	Combined audiological and developmental surveillance improves outcomes in dual-diagnosed children.

Prenatal and Perinatal Factors

The prenatal period is critical for both brain and auditory system development. Disruptions during this time due to infection, maternal illness, or inflammatory processes can result in structural and functional abnormalities that manifest as ASD, hearing impairment, or both. For instance:

1. Maternal diabetes and obesity have been linked to increased ASD risk.
2. Premature birth and low birth weight are associated with a higher likelihood of hearing loss and neurodevelopmental delays.
3. Birth trauma, including prolonged labor or complications involving oxygen deprivation (hypoxic-ischemic injury), may also lead to deficits in auditory processing and neurocognitive functioning.

Furthermore, the presence of multiple risk factors such as genetic susceptibility combined with prenatal infection or toxic exposure can compound the impact, resulting in more severe developmental outcomes and increasing the probability of dual diagnoses.

Implications for Screening and Prevention

Implications for screening and prevention include:

1. Understanding the etiological roles of genetics, environment, and prenatal factors in ASD and hearing impairment underscores the importance of comprehensive early screening, particularly for high-risk populations.
2. Universal newborn hearing screening (UNHS) has already become standard practice in many countries, facilitating the early identification of hearing loss. However, there is a need for parallel early screening for ASD, especially among children with known sensory deficits, to ensure timely detection of co-occurring developmental concerns.
3. Genetic counseling, prenatal care, and public health interventions such as vaccination programs (e.g., for rubella), maternal education, and teratogen avoidance can play key roles in reducing preventable causes of both conditions.
4. Additionally, advances in genomics and epigenetics may eventually allow for more precise risk profiling and personalized early intervention strategies.

Impact on Brain Development and Communication Systems

The co-occurrence of ASD and hearing impairment exerts a significant and multifaceted impact on brain development and communication systems, affecting the way individuals perceive, process, and express information.

Understanding the neurological and functional implications of these dual conditions is critical for designing effective interventions that support language acquisition, cognitive growth, and social participation (Brady et al., 2021).

Effects on Brain Development

Both ASD and hearing impairment independently influence the developing brain, and their co-occurrence can lead to compounded alterations in neural architecture, connectivity, and function.

In ASD, research consistently shows abnormal patterns of brain growth, including early overgrowth in some regions such as the frontal cortex and amygdala, followed by atypical pruning and connectivity. These patterns are often accompanied by reduced integration between brain regions, particularly between those involved in social-emotional processing, executive functioning, and sensory integration. Functional MRI studies have also identified disruptions in the default mode network (DMN) and salience network, which are critical for attention, self-regulation, and social awareness.

In individuals with congenital hearing loss, auditory deprivation leads to significant reorganization of the auditory cortex. When the brain is not stimulated by sound input during critical periods of development, neural circuits in the auditory pathways become underdeveloped or repurposed, a phenomenon known as cross-modal plasticity (Hall & Samar, 2020). In such cases, regions typically responsible for auditory processing may begin to process visual or tactile stimuli instead, which can be adaptive but may also interfere with later auditory rehabilitation (e.g., cochlear implantation).

When ASD and hearing impairment co-occur, these neurodevelopmental disruptions may interact, resulting in greater challenges in multisensory integration, attention, and emotional regulation. Both conditions may affect temporal processing, the brain's ability to interpret the timing of stimuli, making it more difficult to synchronize auditory, visual, and motor information, which is crucial for language and social communication development.

Impact on Communication Systems

The dual impact on communication systems is particularly profound. Language development, whether spoken or signed, relies heavily on early sensory input, social reciprocity, and cognitive-linguistic processing, all areas that may be compromised in individuals with both ASD and hearing loss (Davidson & Quittner, 2020; Rizzolatti & Sinigaglia, 2016).

In ASD, children may show delayed or atypical language development, including challenges in using and understanding pragmatic language, difficulties with joint attention, and echolalia. While some children may be nonverbal, others may develop fluent speech that lacks social appropriateness or emotional nuance (Davidson & Quittner, 2020). Theory of mind deficits and limited use of nonverbal communication cues (e.g., gestures, facial expressions) further impede effective interpersonal communication (Baron-Cohen et al., 2013).

In children with hearing impairment, language delays are commonly attributed to reduced auditory access to linguistic input, particularly in cases of late diagnosis or insufficient amplification. Even with early use of hearing aids or cochlear implants, children may still experience delays in phonological awareness, vocabulary acquisition, and grammar, particularly if they lack consistent exposure to rich language models.

In cases of dual diagnosis, both the neurological differences of ASD and the sensory limitations of hearing impairment contribute to a more complex and heterogeneous communication profile. For example, a child with ASD may have difficulty initiating communication due to social cognition deficits, while hearing loss may limit their ability to perceive environmental sounds or spoken language cues. Some children may not benefit fully from auditory-based communication methods and may require augmentative and alternative communication (AAC) systems or sign language, tailored to their cognitive and sensory strengths (American Speech-Language-Hearing Association, 2021; Schlosser & Koul, 2021).

Moreover, the social use of language, known as pragmatic communication, is particularly affected. Children with dual diagnoses often struggle with turn-taking, topic maintenance, and interpreting body language or tone of voice, especially when auditory and visual signals are unclear or overwhelming. These limitations can lead to social isolation, frustration, and behavioral issues, further affecting academic and emotional development (Brown, L. X. Z. & Ashkenazy, 2021).

Intervention Considerations

Given the intricate interaction between ASD, hearing impairment, and brain development, intervention must be early, individualized, and multidisciplinary. Effective strategies may include:

1. Integrated speech and language therapy, combining auditory-verbal and visual-gestural methods.
2. Use of AAC tools, such as picture exchange systems, speech-generating devices, or signed communication.
3. Parent coaching and training to support responsive communication in natural contexts.
4. Environmental modifications to reduce sensory overload and enhance predictability.
5. Collaborative planning between audiologists, educators, speech-language pathologists, and behavior therapists.

Thence, the combined impact of ASD and hearing loss on brain development and communication systems underscores the need for a holistic, neuroscience-informed approach to diagnosis and intervention. A deeper understanding of these effects enables practitioners to tailor support strategies that honor each child's unique neurodiversity and communication needs, promoting inclusion, autonomy, and lifelong learning (National Center for College Students with Disabilities, 2021; Lindsay & Dockrell, 2020).

It sheds light on both similar and distinct neurobiological processes underlying ASD and HI and how each of the disorders influences brain organization, connectivity, and sensory processing in unique and occasionally overlapping ways. It further identifies three major points – neural basis, mirror neuron system, and neuroplasticity – that interact synergistically to describe the neurodevelopmental interactions of significant complexity that lead to dual diagnosis.

This distinction is based on Neural Basis differences. Abnormal brain connectivity patterns in persons with ASD have been effectively reported and include hyperconnectivity and hypoconnectivity in the cortical and subcortical areas (Uddin et al., 2013). The neuroimaging investigations demonstrate the presence of abnormalities in the default mode network (DMN), salience network, and social brain, including the superior temporal sulcus and amygdala, which is essential in emotional processing and social communication (Just et al., 2012). These neural variations are the cause of difficulties of integrating sensory and social signals leading to distorted perception and behavior.

Conversely, the impaired hearing is mainly in the auditory neural pathways where the impaired auditory stimulation of the critical developmental periods causes the reduction in the activation of the auditory cortex and downstream processing areas (Kral & Sharma, 2012). This sensory loss is able to modify cortical development, which redirects neural resources towards non-auditory modalities. Although ASD neural impairment is caused by inherent neurodevelopmental anomalies, hearing impairment is caused by extrinsic sensory deprivation which causes neural functionality reorganization by compensatory processes.

Another point of convergence as well as divergence is offered by the Mirror Neuron System (MNS). The MNS, which constitutes areas of the inferior

Table 2.4. A brief comparison of shared and distinct neural pathways underlying ASD and Hearing Impairment to support clearer neurodevelopmental understanding

Aspect	*ASD*	*Hearing Impairment*
Neural Basis	Atypical brain connectivity.	Reduced auditory stimulation.
Mirror Neuron System	Underactive.	Limited social-linguistic feedback.
Plasticity	Impaired multisensory integration.	Cross-modal reorganization.

frontal gyrus and inferior parietal lobule is vital in imitation, empathy, and decoding the intentions of others. In ASD, this system is relatively inactive, which restricts the possibility of imitating social behavior and determining the emotional state, thereby influencing social reciprocity (Rizzolatti & Sinigaglia, 2016).

Hearing impaired people are not neurologically predisposed to MNS impairment, but they tend to have limited social-linguistic feedback because of getting less exposure to auditory–verbal communication, particularly when sign language or visual communication is not acquired at a young age. Indirectly this deprivation may limit the activation of MNS because imitation and social cognition require multifaceted multisensory interaction between caregivers and peers.

Hence, the two groups can exhibit social-emotional learning deficits, but via different developmental mechanisms, namely: neurological in ASD; and environmental in hearing loss.

The two conditions have a significant difference in neuroplasticity. In ASD, unusual processing of sensory information is marked by inability to integrate and interpret data of various sensory modalities (Marco et al., 2011). This deficiency causes hypersensitivity or hyposensitivity in any of the senses, which is part of behavior rigidity and non-interactional lives. On the contrary, the hearing impairment usually results in cross-modal reorganization when the auditory brain area becomes re-purposed to receive visual or tactile impressions, which is already evidence of the amazing adaptability of the brain (Lomber et al., 2010). This compensatory re-organization improves visual–spatial awareness and lip-reading capacity but can also make it more difficult to use auditory rehabilitation therapy after cochlear implantation because cortical pathways have already been re-organized towards non-auditory input.

These patterns combine to indicate that both ASD and hearing impairment share the fact that both senses and neural integration is altered, but the causes of these changes are different: ASD is a result of intrinsic developmental differences in connectivity, whereas hearing impairment is an adaptive restructuring of neural circuits due to sensory deprivation. Clinicians and educators need to learn about these differences to implement specific interventions that follow the neurobiological architecture of both conditions and combine auditory habilitation, sensory modulation, and social communications training in one holistic approach to the needs of individuals with dual diagnoses.

It gives a broad description of the multifactorial causes of ASD and hearing impairment (HI), which identifies the differences or similarities between the genetic, environmental, and prenatal factors that lead to their occurrence and comorbidity. These etiological intersections are important to understand in order to develop early diagnosis, genetic counselling, and preventive measures in dual-diagnosis communities (Brookman-Frazee et al., 2006).

The most recurrently recorded causes of both disorders are genetic factors, even though they are manifested in varying biological processes. Transmission

Table 2.5. A brief comparison of genetic, environmental, and prenatal influences contributing to ASD, Hearing Impairment, and their overlapping developmental risks

Factor	*ASD*	*Hearing Impairment*	*Shared Influence*
Genetic	SHANK3, CHD8, MECP2	GJB2, SLC26A4	Chromosomal overlaps (15q, 22q).
Environmental	Toxins, stress.	Noise, infections.	Maternal CMV, rubella.
Prenatal	Advanced parental age.	Ototoxic exposure.	Prematurity, hypoxia.

ancestry in ASD, there is a great deal of genetic predisposition both in isolated cases of de novo mutation and polygenic inheritance. Some of the predominant genes include SHANK3, CHD8, and MECP2, which are involved in the regulation of synapses, neuron signaling, and chromatin remodeling, which play an important role in the neurodevelopment and cognitive integration (De Rubeis & Buxbaum, 2015). The impairment of these genes is linked to abnormal brain connection, deficit on social-communication and repetitive behaviors.

In hearing deafness, genetic etiology has been identified to cause a majority of congenital deafness – most notably GJB2 and SLC26A4, which is involved in the formation of gap junctions and ion transport in the inner ear (Smith et al., 2005). These mutations disrupt the functioning of the cochlear and transmission of the auditory signals. Notably, overlaps between chromosomes (15q11–13 and 22q11–13) have been observed in both ASD and congenital hearing loss, and thus this implicates a common neuro-sensory weakness that obscures conventional diagnostic lines (Harrison et al., 2019). This overlap of loci might contribute to the presence of some syndromic forms whose alleles show an overlapping pattern of both the auditory and neurodevelopmental impairment (e.g., Usher syndrome or 22q11 deletion syndrome).

The environmental factors are also of fundamental importance because they interact with the genetic susceptibility to produce a genetic predisposition, which is epigenetically and teratogenically controlled. In ASD, exposure to environmental toxins (e.g., heavy metals, pesticides, and air pollutants) and maternal stress during pregnancy, as well as some pharmaceutical agents (e.g., valproate), have been linked with the risk (Christensen et al., 2013). The exposures may interfere with the neural development, synaptic maturation, and immune response.

In deafness, environmental factors are commonly chronic exposure to noise, bacterial or virus infection and ototoxic drugs, which directly destroy cochlear structures. Environmental factors that are common – e.g., maternal cytomegalovirus (CMV) and rubella infection – are especially important. The two pathogens are capable of affecting the developing auditory system and manipulating fetal brain development to cause a range of sensory, cognitive, and communication difficulties (Lanzieri et al., 2014). This overlap highlights the role of environmental insults as typical teratogenic pathways affecting auditory and neural spheres of activity in tandem with one another.

These risks are further complicated by the prenatal factors, which act at the border between genetic susceptibility and environmental impact. In ASD, the factors that have been regularly associated with abnormal neurodevelopment and the high prevalence of autism are advanced parental age, maternal metabolic disorder, and inflammatory reactions during pregnancy (Sandin et al., 2016). In the case of hearing impairment, the prenatal exposure to ototoxic agents may be associated with drug ototoxicity (amino glycoside antibiotics or chemotherapy), or the physiological characteristics of the fetus auditory organogenesis (e.g. insufficient ossicles within the middle ear cavity).

Both disorders, though, are combined with a number of perinatal and prenatal stressors increasing the chance of dual diagnosis. Prematurity, low birth weight, and perinatal hypoxia may interfere with the delivery of oxygen and nutrients to the developing brain and auditory system, leading to structural and functional defects. These common prenatal processes help us to underline that dual diagnosis is not always accidental, it is the convergence of a variety of biological and environmental stressors on the developing nervous system.

The etiological environment of ASD and hearing impairment are related instead of separated. The interactions of genetic predispositions, environmental exposures, and prenatal conditions result in overlapping risk paths that determine early sensory and cognitive development. The identification of these common effects supports the idea of combined neonatal screening programs, genetic testing, and maternal health programs. Risk can be minimized and healthier neurodevelopmental outcomes supported by means of early detection and preventive treatment, which can be achieved through vaccination, control of infection, and prevention of toxins and other threats to children at the border of silence and spectrum.

Application to a Real Life Situation: The Comprehension of Sensory Overload

A six-year-old child, Bilal, who was ASD with mild sensorineural hearing impairment, became upset during group activities. Teachers observed that he took off his hearing aids a lot and covered his ears. An occupational therapist determined hypersensitivity to auditory input and touch. The contribution of soft lighting in the classroom, low background noise, and break intervals helped Bilal feel more relaxed and engaged. This case illustrates the importance of sensory modulation and environmental adaptation to decrease stress and improve learning in children with dual sensory-neurodevelopmental difficulties (Duncan & Tangen, 2020).

Summary

1 There are neural dysfunctions between ASD and hearing loss, such as defective connectivity and mirror-neurons variations.
2 There are also specific biological pathways of each condition with ASD being neurodevelopmental and hearing loss mainly sensory.
3 Dual diagnosis changes the sensory integration, which is usually accompanied with auditory deprivation and hypersensitivity.
4 Risk and brain development is combined through the effects of genetic, environmental and prenatal factors.
5 Multisensory and neurodevelopmental views are used to make more individualized interventions.

References

American Speech-Language-Hearing Association. (2021). *Augmentative and alternative communication (AAC)*. https://www.asha.org/practice.

Anderson, S., & Haegele, J. (2023). Neural pathways and social cognition in ASD and hearing impairment. *Journal of Neurodevelopmental Disorders*, 15(2), 45–59. doi:10.1007/s10803-023-05812-4.

Baron-Cohen, S., Ashwin, E., Ashwin, C., Tavassoli, T., & Chakrabarti, B. (2013). The genetics of autism spectrum conditions. *Trends in Cognitive Sciences*, 17(9), 493–500. doi:10.1016/j.tics.2013.08.003.

Brady, N., Stiles, A., & MacDonald, M. (2021). Neurodevelopmental impacts of dual diagnoses: ASD and hearing loss. *Frontiers in Psychology*, 12, 641820. doi:10.3389/fpsyg.2021.641820.

Brookman-Frazee, L., Stahmer, A., Baker-Ericzén, M., & Tsai, K. (2006). Parenting interventions for children with autism spectrum disorders. *Journal of Child and Family Studies*, 15(3), 341–354. doi:10.1007/s10826-006-9026-4.

Brown, L. X. Z., & Ashkenazy, S. (2021). Pragmatic communication deficits in children with ASD and hearing impairment. *Journal of Communication Disorders*, 91, 105–118. doi:10.1016/j.jcomdis.2020.105118.

Buckner, R. L., Andrews-Hanna, J. R., & Schacter, D. L. (2008). The brain's default network: Anatomy, function, and relevance to disease. *Annals of the New York Academy of Sciences, 1124*, 1–38. doi:10.1196/annals.1440.011.

Burke, M. M., & Hodapp, R. M. (2020). Environmental stressors and developmental outcomes in children with sensory impairments. *Developmental Neurorehabilitation*, 23(4), 215–224. doi:10.1080/17518423.2019.1659182.

Christensen, J., Grønborg, T., Sørensen, M. J., Schendel, D., Parner, E. T., Pedersen, L. H., & Vestergaard, M. (2013). Prenatal valproate exposure and risk of autism spectrum disorders and childhood autism. *JAMA*, 309(16), 1696–1703. doi:10.1001/jama.2013.2270.

Davidson, L., & Quittner, A. (2020). Communication outcomes in children with dual sensory and neurodevelopmental disorders. *Ear and Hearing*, 41(6), 1405–1415. doi:10.1097/AUD.0000000000000882.

De Rubeis, S., & Buxbaum, J. D. (2015). Genetics and genomics of autism spectrum disorder: Overview and recent developments. *Current Opinion in Pediatrics*, 27(6), 685–693. doi:10.1097/MOP.0000000000000277.

Duncan, R., & Tangen, J. (2020). Sensory modulation and environmental adaptation in dual-diagnosed children. *Occupational Therapy International, 2020*, 1–10. doi:10.1155/2020/8892345.

Hagerman, R. J., & Hagerman, P. J. (2002). Fragile X syndrome: Diagnosis, treatment, and research. *Pediatric Clinics of North America*, 49(5), 919–929. doi:10.1016/S0031-3955(02)00024–0

Hall, M., & Samar, V. (2020). Auditory deprivation and neural connectivity: Implications for cochlear implantation. *Neuroscience & Biobehavioral Reviews*, 113, 240–252. doi:10.1016/j.neubiorev.2020.03.006.

Harrison, M., Brook, A., & Baker, L. (2019). Chromosomal overlaps in ASD and congenital hearing loss: Genetic insights. *American Journal of Medical Genetics Part C: Seminars in Medical Genetics*, 181(4), 511–523. doi:10.1002/ajmg.c.31703.

Just, M. A., Keller, T. A., Malave, V. L., Kana, R. K., & Varma, S. (2012). Autism as a neural systems disorder: A theory of frontal-posterior underconnectivity. *Neuroscience & Biobehavioral Reviews*, 36(4), 1292–1313. doi:10.1016/j.neubiorev.2012.02.007.

Kral, A., & Sharma, A. (2012). Developmental neuroplasticity after cochlear implantation. *Trends in Neurosciences*, 35(2), 111–122. doi:10.1016/j.tins.2011.11.005.

Lanzieri, T. M., Dollard, S. C., Josephson, C. L., Bialek, S. R., & Cannon, M. J. (2014). Hearing loss in children with congenital cytomegalovirus infection. *Journal of Pediatrics*, 164(5), 1037–1043. doi:10.1016/j.jpeds.2013.12.029.

Lindsay, G., & Dockrell, J. (2020). Educational support for children with ASD and hearing impairment. *International Journal of Inclusive Education*, 24(7), 735–750. doi:10.1080/13603116.2019.1590408.

Lomber, S. G., Meredith, M. A., & Kral, A. (2010). Cross-modal plasticity in specific auditory cortices. *Hearing Research*, 270(1–2),65–72. doi:10.1016/j.heares.2010.08.002.

Marco, E. J., Hinkley, L. B., Hill, S. S., & Nagarajan, S. S. (2011). Sensory processing in autism: A review of neurophysiologic findings. *Pediatric Research*, 69(5 *Pt* 2), 48R–54R. doi:10.1203/PDR.0b013e3182130c54.

National Center for College Students with Disabilities. (2021). *Supporting students with dual sensory-neurodevelopmental disorders in higher education.* https://www.nccsd.org.

Rizzolatti, G., & Sinigaglia, C. (2016). The mirror mechanism: A basic principle of brain function. *Nature Reviews Neuroscience*, 17, 757–765. doi:10.1038/nrn.2016.135.

Sandin, S., Lichtenstein, P., Kuja-Halkola, R., Hultman, C., Larsson, H., & Reichenberg, A. (2016). The heritability of autism spectrum disorder. *JAMA*, 315(1), 68–76. doi:10.1001/jama.2015.17271.

Schlosser, R. W., & Koul, R. (2021). Augmentative and alternative communication interventions for dual-diagnosis children. *Journal of Developmental and Physical Disabilities*, 33, 111–133. doi:10.1007/s10882-020-09815-1.

Smith, R. J. H., Bale, J. F., & White, K. R. (2005). Sensorineural hearing loss in children. *Lancet*, 365(9462), 879–890. doi:10.1016/S0140-6736(05)17911–17917.

Soorya, L., & Tang, K. (2022). Multisensory intervention strategies in dual-diagnosed children. *Journal of Autism and Developmental Disorders*, 52, 4035–4048. doi:10.1007/s10803-021-05233-0.

Uddin, L. Q., Supekar, K., & Menon, V. (2013). Reconceptualizing functional brain connectivity in autism from a developmental perspective. *Frontiers in Human Neuroscience*, 7, 458. doi:10.3389/fnhum.2013.00458.

Chapter 3

Assessment and Diagnostic Challenges in Dual Diagnosis

Tools and Techniques for Differential Diagnosis

The process of diagnosing co-occurring Autism Spectrum Disorder (ASD) and hearing impairment requires precise and thoughtful use of differential diagnostic tools and techniques, as both conditions share overlapping features that can complicate accurate identification. Effective differential diagnosis involves not only distinguishing between ASD and hearing loss but also recognizing when the two conditions coexist. This is essential for developing appropriate intervention plans and optimizing developmental outcomes.

Challenges in Differential Diagnosis

Diagnostic confusion often arises due to similar behavioral manifestations such as limited verbal language, poor eye contact, and difficulties in social interaction. In children with hearing impairment, these behaviors may result from reduced auditory access rather than underlying social-communicative deficits typical of ASD. Conversely, children with ASD who also have undiagnosed hearing loss may not respond to auditory stimuli, leading to the false assumption that autism symptoms are more severe than they actually are.

Therefore, clinicians must rely on a multidimensional and interdisciplinary approach, integrating audiological, developmental, psychological, and behavioral assessments, to accurately distinguish the presence and interaction of both conditions.

Core Tools and Techniques (CTTs)

There are six of these, as follows.

CTT 1: Audiological Evaluation

A comprehensive hearing assessment is the first step in ruling out or confirming hearing loss. This includes:

DOI: 10.4324/9781003750611-3

1 Otoacoustic Emissions (OAE) and Auditory Brainstem Response (ABR) for newborns and young children.
2 Pure tone audiometry, tympanometry, and speech audiometry for older children.

Tests 1 and 2 establish the type (conductive, sensorineural, or mixed) and severity of hearing loss. It is crucial that hearing status be clearly established before assessing for ASD.

CTT 2: Developmental and Behavioral Assessments

Standardized developmental assessments are essential in identifying delays or atypical patterns (Sparrow et al., 2016). Tools commonly used include the following:

1 Bayley Scales of Infant and Toddler Development.
2 Vineland Adaptive Behavior Scales (VABS).
3 Mullen Scales of Early Learning.

These instruments assess domains such as communication, socialization, and motor skills. In children with hearing loss, it is important that assessments account for the child's preferred communication modality (spoken, signed, or augmented).

CTT 3: Autism-Specific Screening Tools

Several established autism screening and diagnostic tools can be adapted for use with deaf or hard of hearing (DHH) children:

1 Autism Diagnostic Observation Schedule, Second Edition (ADOS-2): Though widely used, it may need modification for nonverbal or signing children. Visual schedules and signed instructions can increase accessibility.
2 Modified Checklist for Autism in Toddlers (M-CHAT-R): Can be used for early screening, but interpretation should consider communication mode and developmental history.
3 Diagnostic Interview for Social and Communication Disorders (DISCO) and Autism Diagnostic Interview – Revised (ADI-R): These parent-report instruments can be particularly informative when clinicians are unfamiliar with DHH communication styles.

CTT 4: Specialized Tools for DHH Children

Recognizing the need for culturally and linguistically sensitive instruments, researchers have developed tools specifically for DHH populations, as follows:

1 Social Communication Questionnaire – Deaf Adaptation (SCQ-DA).
2 Autism Spectrum Screening Questionnaire – Deaf Children (ASSQ-DC).

These tools incorporate behavior norms appropriate to deaf culture and visual communication methods, reducing the risk of misdiagnosis (van Gent et al. 2007).

CTT 5: Functional Communication Assessment

A thorough assessment of how the child communicates across contexts is essential. Observations should include structured and unstructured settings, and evaluators should be fluent in the child's communication mode (e.g., American Sign Language, Pakistan Sign Language, or spoken language with amplification). Use of augmentative and alternative communication (AAC) systems should also be explored where relevant (Schlosser & Koul, 2021).

CTT 6: Interdisciplinary Case Reviews

Given the complexity of dual diagnoses, differential diagnosis should be a team-based process involving:

1 Audiologists.
2 Developmental pediatricians.
3 Speech-language pathologists.
4 Special educators.
5 Psychologists with experience in both ASD and hearing impairment.

Case conferences and shared decision-making enable a holistic view of the child's strengths and challenges, avoiding diagnostic overshadowing.

Best Practices in Application

Listed here are the four best practices in application:

1 Modify environments during assessments to reduce sensory distractions.
2 Use visual supports and interpreters or sign-fluent assessors when needed.
3 Prioritize parental input, developmental history, and behavioral patterns across multiple settings.
4 Remain culturally responsive and aware of the child's linguistic background and social context.

Conclusion

Differential diagnosis of ASD and hearing impairment requires methodical, adapted, and culturally informed assessment strategies. The use of specialized tools, interdisciplinary collaboration, and clear understanding of communication modalities ensures more accurate diagnoses, prevents misinterpretation of symptoms, and paves the way for more effective individualized interventions. As research continues to advance, the refinement of diagnostic instruments will further support accurate identification and better outcomes for individuals with complex developmental profiles.

Challenges in Using Standard ASD Diagnostic Tools for DHH Individuals

Diagnosing Autism Spectrum Disorder (ASD) in individuals who are Deaf or Hard of Hearing (DHH) presents distinct and significant challenges. Standard ASD diagnostic tools, such as the Autism Diagnostic Observation Schedule (ADOS), the Autism Diagnostic Interview–Revised (ADI-R), and the Modified Checklist for Autism in Toddlers (M-CHAT-R), were originally developed and normed on typically hearing populations, often without consideration for cultural, linguistic, and sensory differences found in DHH individuals. The inappropriate application of these tools can result in misdiagnosis, underdiagnosis, or overdiagnosis, leading to delayed or ineffective interventions (Lord et al. 2012).

LINGUISTIC AND COMMUNICATION BARRIERS

Many standard ASD tools rely heavily on spoken language and verbal interaction as a means of assessing communication skills. For DHH individuals, particularly those who use sign language, these tools can be linguistically inappropriate. If the evaluator is not fluent in the child's primary mode of communication, whether it be American Sign Language (ASL), Pakistan Sign Language (PSL), or another sign system, key aspects of communicative intent, reciprocity, and language use may be misunderstood or overlooked.

Moreover, signed languages have different grammatical structures and modes of expression than spoken languages. Behaviors such as avoiding eye contact or repeating signs (which may be normal in DHH communication contexts) could be incorrectly interpreted as signs of autism. Conversely, a DHH child's limited expressive language, especially if exposed to language late, may be mistaken for autistic features when they are instead related to language deprivation (Deaf Child Worldwide, 2021).

CULTURAL MISINTERPRETATION OF BEHAVIORS

Many behaviors considered "red flags" for ASD, such as lack of response to name, limited verbal output, or unusual prosody, can occur naturally in DHH children due to auditory limitations or cultural norms within the deaf community. For example:

1 DHH children may not respond to auditory cues, which could be interpreted as inattention.
2 Eye contact norms in deaf culture differ from hearing culture; gaze shifts are part of linguistic communication in sign language but may be perceived as unusual in ASD-focused assessments.

This cultural mismatch can lead clinicians unfamiliar with deaf culture to erroneously pathologize behaviors that are adaptive or typical in DHH contexts.

INACCESSIBILITY OF TEST ITEMS AND FORMATS

Many standardized tools include auditory tasks, verbal instructions, or sound-based cues that are inherently inaccessible to DHH individuals. Even with accommodations, the intent of certain tasks (e.g., responding to the sound of one's name, engaging in pretend play with verbal prompts) may not translate effectively into a visual or tactile modality. This reduces the validity of test scores and may lead to incorrect diagnostic conclusions.

Furthermore, even translated or interpreted versions of assessment tools may not preserve the original meaning or developmental expectations. Assessors using interpreters risk misreading subtle communication behaviors, particularly in assessments that rely on nuanced social-pragmatic cues.

DEVELOPMENTAL IMPACT OF LANGUAGE DEPRIVATION

Many DHH children, especially those born to hearing parents, experience delayed exposure to accessible language, which may cause developmental delays in cognitive, social, and communicative domains (Deaf Child Worldwide, 2021). This early language deprivation can result in behaviors that superficially resemble ASD, such as:

1 Limited joint attention.
2 Delayed theory of mind development.
3 Poor narrative or conversational skills.

Without a careful developmental history and culturally informed assessment, these delays may be misattributed to autism rather than to insufficient early language input.

LACK OF NORMED ASD TOOLS FOR DHH POPULATIONS

Very few ASD diagnostic tools have been adapted or validated for use with DHH individuals. Tools such as the Autism Spectrum Screening Questionnaire – Deaf Children (ASSQ-DC), and the Social Communication

Questionnaire – Deaf Adaptation (SCQ-DA) have emerged to address this gap, but remain under-utilized and not yet widely adopted in clinical settings. The lack of standardized norms for DHH children further complicates the interpretation of diagnostic results (Luterman, 2009).

PROFESSIONAL EXPERTISE GAPS

A significant challenge in using standard ASD diagnostic tools with DHH individuals is the limited availability of professionals trained in both autism and deafness. Without interdisciplinary expertise, diagnostic teams may misinterpret behavior, communication, and developmental milestones, leading to diagnostic overshadowing, where one condition (e.g., hearing loss) masks or overshadows the symptoms of the other (e.g., ASD).

Conclusion and Recommendations

The use of standard ASD diagnostic tools with DHH individuals must be approached with caution, cultural competence, and appropriate adaptations. A valid diagnosis requires:

1. Use of interpreters or assessors fluent in the child's primary language.
2. Selection of modified or adapted tools specifically designed for DHH populations.
3. A developmental history that distinguishes between language deprivation and core autistic traits (Deaf Child Worldwide, 2021).
4. Interdisciplinary collaboration involving audiologists, speech-language pathologists, psychologists, and educators with dual expertise.

In conclusion, accurate diagnosis of ASD in DHH individuals demands culturally responsive, linguistically appropriate, and sensory-aware practices. Only by addressing the inherent limitations of standard tools can we ensure equity in identification, access to services, and long-term developmental support for this uniquely vulnerable population.

Role of Multidisciplinary Teams: Audiology, Psychology, Speech–Language, Special Education

Effective identification, diagnosis, and intervention for individuals with co-occurring ASD and hearing impairment require a multidisciplinary team (MDT) approach. Due to the complex and overlapping nature of both conditions, no single professional discipline can comprehensively assess or address the diverse needs of this population. A collaborative model, drawing expertise from audiology, psychology, speech-language pathology, and special education, ensures that all developmental, sensory, cognitive, communicative, and educational dimensions are considered in the evaluation and support process (Turnbull & Stowe, 2021).

AUDIOLOGY: ASSESSING AND MANAGING AUDITORY FUNCTION

The audiologist plays a foundational role in the MDT by conducting comprehensive hearing assessments to determine the type and degree of hearing loss. This includes:

1 Otoacoustic Emissions (OAE) and Auditory Brainstem Response (ABR) for early identification.
2 Behavioral audiometry and speech discrimination testing for older children.
3 Assessment of hearing aid or cochlear implant benefit, auditory access in various environments, and residual hearing capacity.

In the context of dual diagnosis, the audiologist helps differentiate between auditory processing difficulties due to hearing loss and those due to ASD-related sensory dysfunction. They also guide families and educators on the use of assistive listening devices and create auditory habilitation plans that align with the child's broader developmental needs.

PSYCHOLOGY: BEHAVIORAL AND DEVELOPMENTAL ASSESSMENT

Clinical psychologists, particularly those with expertise in developmental and neuropsychological assessment, contribute significantly to:

1 Evaluating cognitive functioning, executive skills, and adaptive behavior.
2 Conducting autism-specific diagnostic assessments (e.g., ADOS-2, ADI-R), while accounting for sensory and linguistic differences in DHH children.
3 Identifying emotional, behavioral, and social challenges, including anxiety, attention difficulties, and regulation issues.
4 Distinguishing between language deprivation symptoms and core ASD traits (Deaf Child Worldwide, 2021).

Psychologists also play a key role in family counseling, helping caregivers understand the child's profile and supporting them through the emotional and practical implications of dual diagnoses.

SPEECH-LANGUAGE PATHOLOGY: COMMUNICATION AND LANGUAGE SUPPORT

Speech-language pathologists (SLPs) are central to understanding and developing the child's receptive and expressive communication, regardless of whether the child communicates via speech, sign language, or augmentative and alternative communication (AAC) systems (Schlosser & Koul, 2021). Their responsibilities include:

1 Conducting language assessments adapted to the child's communication mode.
2 Supporting the development of pragmatic language and social communication skills, which are often impaired in ASD.
3 Designing individualized communication plans that may involve:
   - signed language (e.g., ASL, PSL)
   - speech therapy for auditory-verbal users, and
   - use of AAC devices or picture exchange systems (PECS).

SLPs also collaborate with audiologists to ensure the child is maximizing auditory input when relevant and support language learning in the presence of auditory or cognitive limitations (Geers & Nicholas, 2020).

SPECIAL EDUCATION: ACADEMIC AND FUNCTIONAL SKILL DEVELOPMENT

Special educators provide essential insights into the child's educational functioning, classroom behavior, and learning style (Turnbull & Stowe, 2021). Their role includes the following.

1 Developing and implementing Individualized Education Programs (IEPs) tailored to the dual needs of ASD and hearing loss (National Center for Learning Disabilities, 2023).
2 Modifying curricula and instructional strategies to accommodate sensory, behavioral, and cognitive differences.
3 Promoting inclusive practices, peer interaction, and social skill development in educational settings.
4 Monitoring academic progress and adaptive skill acquisition across time and settings.

Special educators often serve as coordinators of service delivery, ensuring consistency across home, school, and clinical environments. They are instrumental in integrating therapeutic strategies into everyday learning experiences.

BENEFITS OF A MULTIDISCIPLINARY APPROACH

The collaborative work of these professionals results in four things.

1 Accurate and holistic diagnosis, avoiding misinterpretation of overlapping symptoms.
2 Comprehensive intervention plans that address all developmental domains.

3 Continuity of care, where recommendations are consistent and mutually reinforcing.
4 Family-centered support, where parents receive guidance from multiple perspectives within a unified framework.

CONCLUSION

For children with both ASD and hearing impairment, the integration of audiology, psychology, speech-language pathology, and special education is not optional, it is essential. Each discipline offers a unique lens through which to view the child's abilities and challenges. A well-coordinated multidisciplinary team ensures that interventions are informed, inclusive, and individualized, empowering the child to reach their full potential across communication, social, academic, and behavioral domains.

Culturally and Linguistically Responsive Evaluation Practices

Culturally and linguistically responsive evaluation practices are essential when assessing individuals with a dual diagnosis of ASD and hearing impairment, particularly in diverse populations. Such practices ensure that assessments are fair, accurate, and contextually appropriate, minimizing the risk of misdiagnosis, bias, or exclusion. They acknowledge that culture and language profoundly shape how communication, behavior, and disability are expressed, perceived, and interpreted.

WHY CULTURALLY RESPONSIVE PRACTICES MATTER

Standardized diagnostic tools are typically developed and normed on monolingual, hearing, and majority-culture populations. When used with individuals from deaf culture or linguistic minority backgrounds, these tools may not capture the full range of developmental, social, and communicative competencies. In the context of dual diagnosis, the intersection of disability, language modality (e.g., sign language), and cultural identity can create unique profiles that require sensitive and tailored assessment strategies (Erevelles, 2022).

Failure to apply culturally and linguistically responsive evaluation practices can result in:

1 Overdiagnosis of ASD due to misunderstanding culturally normative behaviors or language differences.
2 Underdiagnosis or missed diagnosis of either ASD or hearing loss due to lack of culturally appropriate tools.
3 Ineffective interventions based on inaccurate assumptions about the child's abilities or needs.

CORE PRINCIPLES OF CULTURALLY AND LINGUISTICALLY RESPONSIVE EVALUATION

Understanding Cultural Contexts Evaluators must recognize that communication norms, social behaviors, and parental expectations vary across cultures. Here are two examples.

1. In Deaf culture, direct eye contact and visual attention are critical components of communication and may differ from hearing cultural norms.
2. Some cultures value nonverbal communication, deference to authority, or reduced emotional expressiveness, which could be misinterpreted as autism traits without cultural context.

Professionals must also be aware of disability stigma, access to services, and historical mistrust of institutions, which can influence how families report behaviors or engage with the evaluation process.

Language Accessibility and Modalities Assessments must be conducted in the child's primary language and mode of communication, whether spoken language, signed language (e.g., ASL, PSL), or a combination. This requires:

1. Use of qualified interpreters fluent in both sign language and the target spoken language.
2. Involvement of evaluators who understand language development in DHH populations and bilingual or bimodal language users (Davidson & Quittner, 2020).
3. Avoiding direct translation of assessment tools without validation, as this may distort meaning or developmental expectations.

For children exposed to multiple languages or communication modes, evaluators must consider typical bilingual/bimodal development patterns to avoid pathologizing language mixing or uneven skills across languages.

Use of Adapted and Validated Tools Whenever possible, evaluators should use assessment instruments adapted for DHH individuals or culturally diverse groups. Examples include:

1. Autism Spectrum Screening Questionnaire – Deaf Children (ASSQ-DC).
2. Social Communication Questionnaire – Deaf Adaptation (SCQ-DA).
3. Culturally adapted versions of the ADOS and other autism diagnostic tools, with visual supports and modified scoring criteria.

These tools are designed to reduce linguistic bias and provide a more accurate measure of social, communicative, and behavioral functioning in diverse populations.

FAMILY AND COMMUNITY INVOLVEMENT

Family members are essential informants in culturally responsive assessments. Evaluators should:

1 Elicit detailed developmental histories that include language exposure, educational background, and cultural beliefs about child development and disability.
2 Use open-ended, respectful, and nonjudgmental questions.
3 Validate families' perspectives and include them as active collaborators in the evaluation process.

In addition, community resources such as deaf mentors, cultural liaisons, or bilingual educators can help bridge cultural gaps and enhance trust.

Bias Awareness and Professional Reflection Evaluators must engage in ongoing self-reflection and bias mitigation. This includes:

1 Recognizing personal assumptions about language, behavior, and disability.
2 Avoiding deficit-based interpretations of differences in communication or behavior.
3 Seeking supervision, consultation, or cultural brokers when working with unfamiliar populations.

Culturally and linguistically responsive evaluation is not an optional enhancement; it is a professional and ethical imperative when assessing children with suspected dual diagnoses of ASD and hearing impairment. By honoring cultural values, ensuring language accessibility, and using adapted tools and collaborative approaches, professionals can promote accurate identification, equitable access to services, and culturally affirming support. These practices are foundational for inclusion, empowerment, and the long-term well-being of children and families from diverse backgrounds.

Table 3.1. Purpose of each tool and adaptations made for Deaf and Hard of Hearing (DHH) children

Tool	*Purpose*	*Adaptation for DHH*
ADOS-2	Observes social and communication behavior.	Use signed instructions, visuals.
M-CHAT-R	Early autism screening.	Interpret in context of hearing level.
ASSQ-DC	Screening for DHH children.	Designed for Deaf populations.

This section reviews the main diagnostic tools used for ASD and discusses the necessary modifications required to make these tools valid, culturally relevant, and linguistically accessible for Deaf and Hard of Hearing (DHH) populations. Adapted instruments such as the Autism Diagnostic Observation Schedule-Second Edition (ADOS-2), the Modified Checklist for Autism in Toddlers-Revised (M-CHAT-R), and the Autism Spectrum Screening Questionnaire for Deaf Children (ASSQ-DC) demonstrate that traditional autism assessments, when used without adaptation, may yield inaccurate or inconclusive results for DHH individuals. Inclusion of adapted instruments like the Autism Diagnostic Observation Schedule-Second Edition (ADOS-2), the Modified Checklist for Autism in Toddlers-Revised (M-CHAT-R), and the Autism Spectrum Screening Questionnaire-Deaf Children (ASSQ-DC) represents an effective acknowledgment that traditional autism tools when utilized in their purest forms tend to give inaccurate or inconclusive information regarding DHH populations.

The ADOS-2 is the gold standard non-interview assessment tool of the social communication, interaction, and limited or stereotypical behaviors related to ASD (Lord et al., 2012). Nevertheless, its initial form presupposes the use of verbal communication and responsiveness to sound, which makes it partially inaccessible to the children who can base their communication on visual or signs-based communication. In order to have diagnostic fairness, adaptations made encompass the use of signed instructions, visual cues, and other nonverbal tasks that involve joint attention, use of gestures, and imitations in the signing environment. The examiners, too, have to be proficient in sign language or collaborate with a trained interpreter who is knowledgeable about the specifics of DHH communication. These kinds of adaptations retain the behavioral validity of the tools and reduce the chances of over-attributing sensory or linguistic variability to autism-based deficit. ADOS-2 modules must be applied in a flexible way by allowing bilingual or bimodal communicators to provide answers to questions in both spoken and signed languages, which demonstrate true communicative competence (Shield & Meier, 2020).

The M-CHAT-R is an early childhood developmental screening tool that is used to screen autistic characteristics in toddlers aged 16–30 months. It is highly generalized in its parent-report format and therefore can be very useful in early intervention environments. Nevertheless, the analysis of the results must be interpreted with caution with regard to DHH children. A wide range of red flag symptoms, including inability to respond to name, lack of verbal productions, or lack of social reciprocity, can be the result of hearing impairment and not the difference in neurodevelopment (Deaf Child Worldwide, 2021). Consequently, examiners are required to analyse the responses according to the level at which the child can hear, the availability of amplification, and the exposure to the available language (e.g., sign or total communication). Audiological results and developmental backgrounds should be added to parent interviews in order to separate sensorineural deprivation effects and autistic traits. Placing M-CHAT-R results in the context of the senses can minimize the chances of false positives and enhance over-the-counter sensitivity of the first-line diagnosis of autism in children with hearing impairment.

The ASSQ-DC (Autism Spectrum Screening Questionnaire-Deaf Children) is an important step in the right direction in terms of culturally and linguistically sensitive assessment. The ASSQ-DC is created to address the needs of DHH communities specifically and includes visual communication norms, deaf-specific culture behaviors, along with modified scoring standards (van Gent et al., 2007). This screening instrument is sensitive to the fact that patterns of social interaction, eye gazes, and facial expressions, which are mistakenly thought of in conventional instruments, can have a different meaning in deaf communities. The ASSQ-DC therefore offers a more reliable way of measuring ASD traits in the DHH children without taking into consideration deaf identity cultural uniqueness. The fact that it has been included in diagnostic protocols is an example of a paradigm shift of the deficit-based approaches interpretations to the neurodiversity-affirming and sensory-conscious assessment approaches.

Taken together, Table 3.1 highlights the idea that the correct diagnosis of ASD in DHH children cannot be achieved by mere translation, but it must be conceptually modified to agree with the impact of sensory, linguistic, and cultural realities of a particular child. The standardized diagnostic practices need to be reorganized so that the communication modality (spoken, signed, or multimodal) should be considered as one of the primary variables instead of a confounder. The diagnostic integrity requires interdisciplinary cooperation between audiologists, psychologists, speech-language pathologists, and sign-fluent clinicians. Finally, these modified instruments will not only make it more precise but also reflect the moral necessity of equity, which does not allow silence, difference, or cultural identity to become an impediment to proper understanding and timely assistance.

Table 3.2 outlines the primary roles of each professional in a multidisciplinary team, highlighting the collaborative functions necessary to assess and support children with co-occurring ASD and hearing impairment.

The collaborative functions of professionals in a multidisciplinary team (MDT) are essential for the assessment and support of individuals with co-occurring ASD and hearing impairment, as no single profession alone has the expertise to address the overlapping sensory, communicative, and behavioral

Table 3.2. **Primary roles of professionals, including Audiologist, Psychologist, SLP, and Special Educator, in assessment and intervention**

Professional	*Primary Role*
Audiologist	Assess hearing levels and auditory processing.
Psychologist	Evaluate cognition, behavior, and social-emotional domains.
SLP	Assess speech, sign, or AAC communication.
Special Educator	Integrate interventions in educational setting.

complexities of dual diagnosis. This is due to the fact because of the overlapping sensory, communicative, and behavioral complexities that are in the dual diagnosis, no single profession has the expertise needed to diagnose and interfere with the diagnosis and/or effectively. Rather, a comprehensive and interdisciplinary model, which is based on audiology, psychology, speech-language pathology (SLP), and special education, is necessary to ensure that the specific neurodevelopmental, sensory, and communicative needs of the child are advocated (Turnbull & Stowe, 2021).

The Audiologist is the backbone of the team since he or she evaluates the hearing thresholds, auditory processing capabilities, and amplification outcomes. Their work entails, among other things, objective testing, which includes Otoacoustic Emissions (OAE) and Auditory Brainstem Response (ABR) testing in childhood, and behavioral audiometry and testing speech perception in older children. In addition to detection, audiologists oversee the functional use of assistive listening systems, hearing aids, and cochlear implants, and that children have the best auditory access to the assessments and education. In the cases of dual diagnosis, audiologists work together with other professionals to distinguish between auditory inattention based on hearing loss and social withdrawal that is typical of ASD. They also participate in designing the auditory habilitation programs that are specific to the sensory and cognitive profile of the child (Kral & Sharma, 2012).

The Psychologist has a key role to play in the assessment of cognitive, behavioral, and social-emotional domains underlying learning as well as adaptive functioning. These encompass standardized tests of intellectual quotient, executive functioning, and emotional control and specific tests of autism such as the ADOS-2 or the ADI-R, which can be necessary to adapt to DHH people (Lord et al., 2012). Psychologists also have the role of diagnosing comorbid behavioral disorders, e.g. anxiety, attention deficit or emotional dysregulation that commonly accompany dual diagnoses. Notably, their interpretive paradigm should be able to differentiate between behaviors that result due to language deprivation or sensory access problems and those that result due to neurodevelopmental deviation. Using family counseling and psychoeducation, psychologists also assist parents in learning about the developmental profile of their child and changing the expectations and strategies accordingly.

The communication specialist in the team is the Speech–Language Pathologist (SLP), who deals with expressive and receptive language, both verbal and non-verbal, through supported and non-supported mediums. During dual diagnosis, the area that the SLP is able to address is not only speech but also sign language, augmentative, and alternative communication (AAC) systems as well as pragmatic language usage. Evaluations need to take into account the primary communication mode of the child, which can be spoken, signed, or multimodal and assess competence in that system instead of through the prism of speech only (Schlosser & Koul, 2021). Depending on the needs of each person, SLPs choose personal strategies that can consist of auditory–verbal therapy, sign-supported speech, or AAC interventions, so that the processing of information is functional, reachable, and socially significant. They also work in partnership with educators who help them incorporate the communication supports into their day-to-day life and audiologists who help to maximize their listening conditions.

The Special Educator acts as a mediator between clinical knowledge and education practice, which makes sure that interventions are effectively applied in the educational context. They are mainly tasked with creating and overseeing the Individualized Education Programs (IEPs) that would target the cognitive, social, behavioral, and communication objectives at the same time (National Center for Learning Disabilities, 2023). To meet the learning requirements of learners with autism, special educators modify curricula, develop multisensory instruction plans, and use visual aids to support both auditory deficits and autism. Additionally, they also mediate communication between all team members and families, making it consistent on both clinical and classroom backgrounds. They facilitate peer interaction, self-regulation, and social participation through inclusive pedagogy and thus, translate diagnostic findings into a daily educational success (Brown & Ashkenazy, 2021).

Together, the summarized roles in Table 3.2 represent an interdisciplinary ecosystem of care, in which each professional has their own view of the child but a single understanding is present. Access to sound is facilitated by the audiologist, cognition and behavior are interpreted by the psychologist, communicative competence is determined by the SLP, and functional learning and participation is achieved through the combination of these components by the special educator. These types of collaboration reduce diagnostic overshadowing, increase the coherence of interventions, and promote a holistic development trajectory. Finally, the MDT model supports once again the fact that only joint knowledge, organized activity, and integrated vision can result in the correct assessment of children with ASD and hearing impairment and the provision of meaningful support to them.

Hypothesis: The Strength of Interdisciplinary Assessment

Rida is a five-year-old who made minimal gestures, and was referred to have an evaluation of autism carried out. Her verbal response was not provided during testing, thus raising concerns over severe ASD. The reassessment of her was done by a multidisciplinary team that consisted of an audiologist, a psychologist, and a sign-proficient SLP. Auditory assessment revealed a moderate case of conductive hearing loss, and adaptations on ADOS using visuals indicated the development of joint attention. The team reached a conclusion of dual diagnosis and began a mixed approach to communication. This situation underscores the fact that teamwork is avoiding diagnostic overshadowing and enabling correct identification.

Summary

1. The huge overlap of ASD and hearing loss can result in a misdiagnosis and a lateral delay in support.
2. Deaf/Hard-of-Hearing populations are better served by adapted assessment tools (e.g., SCQ-DA, ASSQ-DC).
3. There should be multidisciplinary cooperation between audiologists, psychologists, SLPs and special educators.
4. Assessments should be language and culturally sensitive, which is based on the mode of communication of the child.
5. Naturalistic observations and insights of families enhance the reliability and accuracy of diagnosis.

References

Brown, C., & Ashkenazy, J. (2021). *Inclusive practices in special education: Strategies for supporting learners with complex needs*. Routledge.

Davidson, K., & Quittner, A. L. (2020). *Language development and assessment in deaf and hard-of-hearing children*. Plural Publishing.

Deaf Child Worldwide. (2021). *Supporting deaf children with developmental differences*. https://deafchildworldwide.org.

Erevelles, N. (2022). *Disability and difference in global contexts: Enabling equitable assessment practices*. Routledge.

Geers, A. E., & Nicholas, J. G. (2020). *Auditory-verbal intervention for children with hearing loss: Foundations and evidence*. Plural Publishing.

Kral, A., & Sharma, A. (2012). Developmental neuroplasticity after cochlear implantation. *Trends in Neurosciences*, 35(2), 111–122. doi:10.1016/j.tins.2011.12.008.

Lord, C., Risi, S., Lambrecht, L., Cook, E. H., Leventhal, B. L., DiLavore, P. C., Pickles, A., & Rutter, M. (2012). *The autism diagnostic observation schedule–second edition (ADOS-2) manual (Part I: Modules 1–4)*. Western Psychological Services.

Luterman, D. (2009). *Counseling persons with communication disorders and their families* (5th ed.). Pro-Ed.

National Center for Learning Disabilities. (2023). *Supporting students with dual diagnoses: Guidelines for individualized education programs*. https://www.ncld.org.

Schlosser, R. W., & Koul, R. (2021). *Augmentative and alternative communication assessment and intervention: Evidence-based practices*. Brookes Publishing.

Shield, A., & Meier, R. P. (2020). *Deaf children and autism: A guide for professionals*. Oxford University Press.

Sparrow, S. S., Cicchetti, D. V., & Saulnier, C. A. (2016). *Vineland adaptive behavior scales* (3rd ed.). Pearson.

Turnbull, A., & Stowe, M. J. (2021). *Multidisciplinary approaches in special education: Coordination and collaboration for complex learners*. Routledge.

van Gent, T., Goedhart, A., Hindley, P., & Treffers, P. (2007). Screening for autism spectrum disorders in deaf children. *Journal of Autism and Developmental Disorders*, 37(2), 208–219. doi:10.1007/s10803-006-0156-7.

Chapter 4

Communication and Language Development Across Modalities

Speech, Sign Language, and Augmentative/Alternative Communication (AAC)

Communication is a central developmental domain profoundly affected in individuals with dual diagnoses of ASD and hearing impairment. These individuals often experience complex challenges in expressive and receptive communication due to the interaction of auditory limitations, social-pragmatic difficulties, and, in many cases, cognitive or behavioral delays. Supporting communication in this population requires a flexible, multimodal approach that includes spoken language, sign language, and augmentative and alternative communication (AAC) systems, used either separately or in combination, to meet each individual's unique needs (Schlosser & Koul, 2021).

Spoken Language: Opportunities and Limitations

Spoken language remains the dominant mode of communication in most educational and social settings. For children with hearing impairment, access to spoken language depends heavily on:

1. Degree and type of hearing loss.
2. Early identification and amplification (e.g., hearing aids, cochlear implants).
3. Consistent language-rich environments.
4. Quality of auditory-verbal therapy and intervention.

When ASD is also present, additional challenges emerge. Many children with ASD may show:

1. Delayed speech or language regression.
2. Echolalia (repetition of words or phrases).
3. Difficulties with prosody, articulation, and expressive clarity.
4. Impairments in pragmatic language use, such as initiating conversation, turn-taking, or understanding figurative language.

DOI: 10.4324/9781003750611-4

For some individuals, spoken language may develop functionally with support; for others, alternative modes of communication may be more effective and less frustrating.

Sign Language: A Visual and Accessible Modality

Sign language (e.g., American Sign Language [ASL], Pakistan Sign Language [PSL], British

Sign Language [BSL]) is a fully developed natural language with its own grammar, structure, and cultural context. It provides a visually accessible mode of communication for individuals who are deaf or hard of hearing, especially those for whom spoken language is not viable or reliable.

For children with ASD and hearing impairment, sign language can offer:

1 A concrete, visual representation of language, which may align with ASD learning styles.
2 Reduced reliance on auditory processing, which can be overwhelming for some.
3 A tool for early language development, particularly in pre-verbal or minimally verbal children.

However, challenges may arise due to the social and motor demands of sign language. Some children with ASD may:

1 Struggle with joint attention, facial expressions, and eye gaze.
2 Have difficulties with fine motor coordination, affecting sign production.
3 Exhibit limited motivation for social interaction, a key component of communicative exchanges in sign.

Despite these challenges, exposure to sign language early, particularly in deaf families or inclusive environments, can enhance language access and social engagement.

The Development of Language and Thought After Cochlear Implants

Cochlear implantation (CI) is one of the greatest achievements in auditory rehabilitation of children with hearing loss, as well as those who have other developmental disorders such asASD. A cochlear implant is connected to the inner ear bypassing the damaged tissue and instead stimulates the auditory nerve directly, giving access to sound and encouraging auditory-verbal learning (Geers & Nicholas, 2020). Nevertheless, there are significant differences in outcomes of language and cognitive development with regard to age at the time of implantation, the level of cognitive ability, environmental stimulation, and co-morbid neurodevelopmental disorders.

Table 4.1. Definition, benefits, cognitive, social-emotional, motor, environmental, and educational implications of sign language for children with ASD and Hearing Impairment, including recommended adaptations and overall impact

Aspect	*Details*
Definition	A natural visual-manual language (e.g., ASL, PSL, BSL) with its own grammar, structure, and cultural identity, used by deaf and hard-of-hearing individuals.
Benefits for ASD + HI	Visual representation aligns with visual learning preferences in ASD. Minimizes auditory processing load. Facilitates early language acquisition for pre-verbal or minimally verbal children.
Cognitive Accessibility	Concrete and visual modality supports language understanding. Can reduce frustration from communication barriers.
Social-Emotional Support	Can promote joint attention and social engagement if introduced early and modeled consistently.
Motor and Social Challenges	Children with ASD may face: 1. Difficulties with eye contact and facial expression. 2. Limited fine motor skills for accurate sign production. 3. Low motivation for social reciprocity.
Environmental Influence	Deaf family exposure or inclusive educational settings enhance sign language acquisition and communication use.
Educational Implications	Teachers and caregivers need training in sign language. Use of visual supports (e.g., picture schedules, gestures) to complement sign.
Adaptations and Supports	Simplified or modified signs. Use of augmentative and alternative communication (AAC) alongside sign. Peer modeling and visual reinforcement.
Overall Impact	Enhances language access, communication, and inclusion for children with dual diagnosis, especially when introduced early.

Language Development following Cochlear Implant

The prevention of early implantation, preferably prior to the age of two, is linked to better results in the understanding and expression of spoken language (Nicholas & Geers, 2018). Children that are provided with CIs at the sensitive age of auditory development exhibits quick improvement in:

1. Phonological awareness and speech intelligibility.
2. Syntactic development and vocabulary development.
3. Better language receptiveness and expressiveness, especially through regular auditory-verbal treatment and enhanced linguistic exposure.

The language outcomes of children with ASD are more diverse. Others show large improvements in receptive vocabulary and communicative intent, and some may still need visual or augmentative support. Both regular intervention of speech-language pathologists, routines, and parent-median communication programs improve progress.

Auditory Processing and Cognitive Development

Cognitive improvement after cochlear implantation is more than just a speech and language improvement. The studies have shown enhancements in:

1 Dual processes of auditory attention and working memory (Kral & Sharma, 2012).
2 Executive functions, the inhibition, cognitive flexibility, and planning (Harris et al., 2021).
3 Theory of mind and social cognition, which is made possible by more access to auditory-social cues.

Nevertheless, children who have dual diagnosis (ASD and hearing impairment) might have a slower improvement in the high-order cognitive domains. This is because there is a similar deficit in sensory integration, joint attention, and symbolic understanding. The interventions are supposed to be a combination of auditory habilitation and structured cognitive-behavioral supports and multimodal communication systems.

Factors Influencing Outcomes

Important predictors of post-implant language and cognitive development are:

1 Implantation (younger = superior neural plasticity).
2 Quality and duration of auditory training.
3 Family interventions and language culture.
4 Stability of device usage and technical service.
5 Co-occurrence of neurodevelopmental disorders.

Bilingualism environments in the form of bimodal (spoken + sign language) have turned out to be helpful in making cognitive flexibility and identity development, as well as in cases where speech cannot be fully understood (Davidson, 2020).

Educational and Therapeutic Consequences

To achieve the best results, the intervention teams ought to:

1. Combine auditory-verbal therapy and visual language aids.
2. Offer continuous cognitive and language tests after implantation.
3. Promote family-based training to maintain communication and the use of the device.
4. Use multimodal instructions, such as AAC, in children with ASD characteristics.

Conclusion

Cochlear implantation is capable of considerably increasing access to auditory functions and contributing to language and cognitive development. Nevertheless, in children with ASD or other developmental disorders, personal and multimodal and interdisciplinary interventions are of utmost importance to achieve the most out of communicative and cognitive possibilities.

Augmentative and Alternative Communication (AAC)

Bridging Gaps in Expression AAC systems encompass a broad range of strategies and tools that support or replace spoken or signed communication (Schlosser & Koul, 2021). These include:

1. Low-tech AAC: Picture Exchange Communication System (PECS), communication boards, visual schedules.
2. High-tech AAC: Speech-generating devices (SGDs), tablet-based apps with symbol or text output (e.g., Proloquo2Go).

AAC is often essential for children with dual diagnoses who are:

1. Nonverbal or minimally verbal.
2. Unable to use speech or sign consistently.
3. In need of visual support to reduce anxiety and support expressive or receptive language.

AAC offers multiple benefits, including:

1. Reducing frustration and behavior issues by providing an immediate communication outlet.
2. Enhancing independence, choice-making, and participation in daily activities.
3. Serving as a bridge to verbal or signed communication with appropriate intervention.

Importantly, research shows that AAC use does not hinder the development of speech or sign; instead, it often facilitates it by strengthening symbolic understanding and communicative intent.

Table 4.2. Key aspects and impacts of sign language for children with ASD and Hearing Impairment, including definition, benefits, cognitive, social-emotional, motor, environmental, educational implications, and adaptations

Aspect	*Details*
Definition	A range of strategies and tools that support or replace spoken or signed communication, enabling individuals to express themselves effectively.
Types of AAC	Low-tech: PECS, communication boards, visual schedules. High-tech: Speech-generating devices (SGDs), apps like Proloquo2Go.
Target Population	Nonverbal or minimally verbal children. Inconsistent speech or sign users. Individuals needing visual support for comprehension and expression.
Benefits	Reduces communication frustration and behavioral challenges. Enhances autonomy and participation. Supports language development and symbolic understanding.
Role in Dual Diagnosis	Serves as a bridge for communication where both speech and sign are limited. Visual tools align with learning preferences and reduce cognitive load.
Integration with Other Supports	Can complement speech therapy, sign language, and visual learning strategies. Customizable to suit individual needs and contexts.
Common Myths	Myth: AAC prevents speech or sign development. Reality: AAC often facilitates speech/sign by reinforcing communicative intent.
Educational Implications	Requires staff training and individualized planning. Should be embedded across settings (home, school, therapy).
Best Practices	Early introduction. Consistent modeling by adults. Multimodal communication approach (speech, sign, AAC used together).

Multimodal Communication: An Individualized Approach

For many individuals with ASD and hearing impairment, no single communication method is sufficient. Instead, a multimodal approach is often most effective, combining spoken language (with amplification), sign language, and AAC based on:

1 Cognitive ability and learning style.
2 Language exposure history.
3 Family and educational support.
4 Sensory sensitivities and preferences.

Professionals should prioritize the development of functional communication, enabling the child to express needs, make choices, engage socially, and participate academically, rather than focusing on one modality exclusively.

Role of Family and Educational Environment

The success of any communication approach is significantly influenced by family involvement, consistency across settings, and staff training. Families and educators must receive the following:

1. Training in the chosen communication systems (sign language classes, AAC use).
2. Support to reinforce communication across daily routines.
3. Guidance in creating language-rich environments adapted to the child's abilities.

Collaborative planning among speech-language pathologists, special educators, audiologists, family members, and paraeducators ensures that the chosen communication modalities are accessible, consistent, and meaningful (Giangreco, 2021).

Conclusion

In individuals with co-occurring ASD and hearing impairment, communication support must be flexible, individualized, and multimodal. Whether using speech, sign language, AAC, or a combination, the ultimate goal is to empower the individual to connect with others, express themselves, and engage meaningfully with their environment. Early and ongoing assessment, interdisciplinary collaboration, and family-centered planning are critical for building effective, functional communication systems that grow with the learner (Shield & Meier, 2020).

Pragmatic Language Deficits and Social Communication Issues

Pragmatic language refers to the use of language in social contexts, the ability to use language appropriately for different purposes, in different settings, and with different conversational partners. It includes skills such as turn-taking, maintaining topics, using appropriate gestures or facial expressions, understanding figurative language, and interpreting others' intentions. In individuals with a dual diagnosis of ASD and hearing impairment, pragmatic language deficits and social communication issues are particularly prominent and multifaceted, often leading to substantial challenges in social interaction and relationship-building.

Pragmatic Language and ASD

Deficits in social-pragmatic communication are one of the core features of ASD, regardless of an individual's verbal ability. Children and adults with ASD may:

1 Have difficulty initiating or sustaining conversations.
2 Use unusual or repetitive language (e.g., echolalia or idiosyncratic phrases).
3 Fail to use or interpret nonverbal cues such as gestures, facial expressions, and tone of voice.
4 Struggle with perspective-taking and understanding social rules (e.g., interrupting, talking too loudly or off-topic).
5 Exhibit limited imaginative play or symbolic use of language.

Even when structural language (vocabulary and grammar) is intact, the functional use of language in social contexts can be significantly impaired.

Impact of hearing impairment on Pragmatic Language

Hearing impairment can further affect pragmatic language development (Davidson & Quittner, 2020), even in individuals without ASD. Children who are deaf or hard of hearing (DHH), particularly those with delayed access to language input, often experience:

1 Reduced exposure to conversational models, limiting opportunities to observe and internalize pragmatic norms.
2 Difficulty overhearing incidental social exchanges, which are critical for learning how language functions in everyday life.
3 Challenges in understanding prosodic features (e.g., intonation, emphasis), which convey emotion and intent.
4 Gaps in learning figurative language, humor, and idioms, especially in spoken language environments.

For DHH children who use sign language, the acquisition of pragmatic skills may be more robust if they are exposed early to fluent signers, such as deaf parents or teachers (Shield & Meier, 2020). However, DHH children raised in environments with limited or inconsistent language models may exhibit pragmatic deficits similar to those seen in ASD (Glickman & Hall, 2021).

Table 4.3. Challenges in conversational skills, nonverbal communication, social reciprocity, figurative language, perspective-taking, symbolic language, prosody, and exposure to language models for children with ASD, Hearing Impairment, and their combined impact in dual diagnosis, along with recommended support strategies

Aspect	*Autism Spectrum Disorder*	*Hearing Impairment*	*Combined Impact in Dual Diagnosis (ASD + HI)*
Conversational Skills	Difficulty initiating/ sustaining conversations. Tendency for monologues or tangents.	Limited exposure to conversational norms. Reduced access to incidental learning.	Severe impairments in initiating/ maintaining dialogue due to compounded barriers.
Nonverbal Communication	Challenges in using/interpreting gestures, facial expressions, eye contact.	Difficulty perceiving auditory cues. Some may rely more heavily on visual cues.	May miss or misinterpret both verbal and nonverbal social cues.
Turn-Taking and Topic Maintenance	Interruptions, off-topic remarks, poor reciprocity.	Limited practice in naturalistic dialogue situations.	Marked struggle with turn-taking and topic shifts, even in structured settings.
Understanding Social Rules	Difficulty with social conventions (e.g., personal space, volume control).	May not overhear or learn implicit rules through observation.	Needs explicit instruction and structured practice for social norms.
Use of Figurative Language	Literal interpretations. difficulty with metaphors, sarcasm, humor.	Delayed comprehension of idioms and abstract language.	Pronounced difficulty in decoding and using figurative or inferential language.
Perspective-Taking (Theory of Mind)	Struggles to infer others' beliefs, intentions, or emotions.	May not access subtle cues indicating mental states of others.	Dual barriers to developing perspective-taking and empathetic communication.
Symbolic/Imaginative Language Use	Limited imaginative play and symbolic language.	Symbolic play may be underdeveloped in absence of rich language models.	Restricted use of imaginative language. May affect narrative and pretend play.

Aspect	*Autism Spectrum Disorder*	*Hearing Impairment*	*Combined Impact in Dual Diagnosis (ASD + HI)*
Prosody and Emotional Tone	Flat or unusual intonation. Inappropriate affect.	Difficulty hearing or producing prosodic cues.	Atypical or absent prosody. Emotional intent may be hard to perceive or convey.
Exposure to Language Models	Social isolation may limit peer interaction and language modelling.	Misses out on overheard social language and incidental learning.	Extremely limited natural exposure. Requires structured modeling and teaching.
Support Strategies Needed	Social communication interventions, visual supports, social stories.	Early access to language (spoken or sign), speech/ language therapy.	Multimodal communication approaches. Integrated AAC, visual schedules, and social-pragmatic instruction.

Dual Diagnosis: ASD and hearing impairment

When ASD and hearing impairment co-occur, the pragmatic and social communication difficulties are often compounded, creating a more complex and severe profile (Brady et al., 2021). These may include:

1 Limited initiation of communication, whether verbal or signed.
2 Poor use of facial expressions and eye gaze, which are critical in both spoken and signed communication.
3 Difficulty adapting communication styles to different people or settings.
4 Challenges in repairing communication breakdowns or recognizing when a message is misunderstood.
5 Literal interpretation of language, with difficulty understanding jokes, sarcasm, or abstract concepts.

Moreover, both ASD and hearing loss can lead to social isolation, which limits opportunities for social-pragmatic development. Children with a dual diagnosis may have fewer peer interactions, reduced motivation for social engagement, or frustration stemming from communication breakdowns.

Assessment Considerations

Standardized tests may not adequately capture pragmatic deficits in children with dual diagnoses. Assessment must include the following:

1 Naturalistic observations across settings (home, school, play).

2 Parent and teacher interviews (e.g., using tools like the Children's Communication Checklist or the Social Communication Questionnaire).
3 Consideration of the child's primary language or modality (spoken, signed, AAC).

Assessors must distinguish between delays due to language deprivation (common in DHH populations) and inherent social-pragmatic deficits related to ASD (Deaf Child Worldwide, 2021).

Intervention Strategies

Addressing pragmatic language deficits and social communication issues requires early, multimodal, and individualized intervention. Key strategies include:

1 Social skills training using structured and naturalistic teaching.
2 Visual supports and scripts to guide interactions and promote generalization.
3 Peer-mediated interventions that facilitate inclusive social experiences (Thiemann-Bourque & Brady, 2021).
4 Use of video modeling, role-playing, and social stories to teach abstract or nuanced skills.
5 Incorporating speech-language therapy and sign language instruction based on the child's strengths and needs (Shield & Meier, 2020).
6 Ensuring that AAC systems are designed to support not just basic requests but also social interactions (e.g., greetings, comments, questions).

Family and school involvement is critical. Caregivers and teachers must model appropriate communication, provide opportunities for structured and unstructured social practice, and reinforce successful social interactions.

Conclusion

Pragmatic language and social communication are areas of significant vulnerability for individuals with co-occurring ASD and hearing impairment. These deficits can profoundly impact peer relationships, academic success, and emotional well-being. By combining culturally responsive assessment with individualized, multimodal intervention strategies, professionals can help foster more meaningful and functional communication, supporting the development of social competence and lifelong interpersonal skills.

Visual Language Strategies for Children with Dual Diagnosis

Children with a dual diagnosis of ASD and hearing impairment present a unique communication profile that benefits greatly from visual language strategies. These strategies leverage the child's strengths in visual learning and provide accessible, consistent modes of communication that do not rely on auditory input or complex social cues. For many children in this population, visual language approaches not only support expressive and receptive communication but also help reduce behavioral frustration, enhance learning, and facilitate social engagement.

Key Visual Language Strategies

Sign Language

For many deaf or hard-of-hearing (DHH) children, natural sign languages such as American Sign Language (ASL), Pakistan Sign Language (PSL), or British Sign Language (BSL) offer a fully accessible linguistic system (Shield & Meier, 2020). When used consistently in the home and educational environments:

1. Sign language can foster early language acquisition.
2. It provides visual-spatial grammar, which is well-suited to children with strong visual memory.
3. Signs can be paired with pictures or gestures for children with ASD who may need additional supports.

For children with ASD, however, challenges may include limited imitation skills, motor planning difficulties, or reduced social motivation to communicate. Therefore, sign language should be introduced using structured, repetitive, and motivating activities, with modeling from fluent users (Shield & Meier, 2020).

Picture Exchange Communication System (PECS)

PECS is a widely used low-tech augmentative communication system that teaches children to initiate communication using pictures. It is especially useful for nonverbal or minimally verbal children with ASD and/or hearing loss.

1. PECS begins with basic requests (e.g., "I want juice") and progresses to more complex functions (e.g., commenting, answering questions).
2. It fosters intentional communication and reinforces the cause-effect relationship between symbol use and outcome.
3. PECS is highly visual and can be customized for home, school, and therapy environments.

PECS does not rely on hearing or verbal imitation, making it ideal for dual diagnosis populations. It can be used as a standalone system or alongside spoken or signed language.

Visual Schedules and Timelines

Children with ASD and hearing loss often struggle with transitions, routine changes, and sequencing of events. Visual schedules provide a concrete representation of daily activities, reducing anxiety and increasing predictability (American Association on Intellectual and Developmental Disabilities, 2021).

1. These can include pictures, icons, or real-life photos.
2. Can be static (on a board) or dynamic (using hook-and-loop fastening pieces or mobile apps).
3. Help children understand "first-then" sequences, time concepts, and expectations.

Visual schedules support independence, emotional regulation, and task completion across home and school settings.

Gesture and Natural Visual Cues

Many children with dual diagnosis benefit from simplified, intentional gestures that accompany speech or sign. These include:

1. Pointing, waving, nodding, and other culturally appropriate body movements.
2. Use of facial expressions, which are crucial in sign languages and social-emotional learning.
3. Visual prompts for actions (e.g., holding up a toothbrush to signal brushing time).

Adults should consistently pair gestures with spoken or signed words to reinforce meaning and promote language development.

Video Modeling

Video modeling uses short video clips to demonstrate target behaviors or skills, such as greeting others, completing a task, or requesting help. It is highly effective for children with ASD due to their preference for visual input and structured routines.

1. Videos can feature peers, adults, or the child themselves.
2. Content can be replayed as needed, supporting repetition and generalization.
3. It is particularly useful for teaching social-pragmatic skills and routines.
4. 4. High-Tech AAC with Visual Interfaces.

Devices such as speech-generating tablets (e.g., Proloquo2Go, LAMP Words for Life) offer customizable interfaces with visual symbols. These tools:

1 Enable expressive language for children who cannot use speech or sign.
2 Can be tailored to the child's developmental level, cultural context, and daily vocabulary.
3 Offer options for visual scanning, grid organization, and symbol-text pairing.

Training for both the child and caregivers is essential for successful implementation.

Implementing Visual Language Strategies: Best Practices

1 Consistency: Use the same visual signs, symbols, or routines across environments.
2 Individualization: Select strategies that match the child's cognitive level, sensory profile, and motor abilities.
3 Collaboration: Involve families, educators, therapists, and interpreters in the planning and use of visual tools.
4 Reinforcement and motivation: Pair communication attempts with meaningful outcomes and positive reinforcement.
5 Monitoring and adaptation: Assess the effectiveness of each strategy over time and modify based on the child's progress and preferences.

Conclusion

Visual language strategies are not only compensatory but can be primary tools for empowering children with ASD and hearing impairment to communicate, connect, and participate. Whether through sign language, pictures, gestures, or AAC, these strategies bridge the communication gap, reduce frustration, and promote language growth and social understanding.

Supporting language acquisition in bilingual environments

Language acquisition in children with a dual diagnosis of Autism Spectrum Disorder (ASD) and hearing impairment presents unique challenges and opportunities, especially in bilingual environments that include both spoken and sign languages. For these children, supporting communication development in a bimodal (visual-manual and auditory-oral) context can be highly beneficial, but it requires thoughtful planning, consistency, and collaborative support.

Understanding Bimodal Bilingualism

Bimodal bilingualism refers to the use of two languages across different modalities, typically a spoken language (e.g., Urdu, English) and a sign language (e.g., Pakistan Sign Language [PSL], and American Sign Language [ASL]). In children with hearing impairment, this approach allows for access to both auditory and visual language pathways. When ASD is also present, the benefits of multimodal input can be maximized if the child has individualized supports that consider sensory, cognitive, and behavioral needs.

Children with ASD and hearing loss may:

1. Show preference for visual learning, which supports sign language use.
2. Experience delays in both languages, requiring targeted intervention.
3. Benefit from the structure and repetition inherent in both spoken and signed systems.
4. Struggle with code-switching or language separation, especially if expressive skills are limited.

Despite these challenges, exposure to two accessible languages does not confuse or delay language development; rather, it broadens communicative options and enhances overall cognitive flexibility.

Key Strategies for Supporting Bilingual Language Acquisition

Use Early and with Consistent Exposure

1. Begin language exposure as early as possible, ideally in both modalities.
2. Ensure the child is surrounded by rich, accessible language models in both spoken and signed forms.
3. Consistent exposure helps form strong neural pathways for each language, even in children with developmental delays.

Create Language-Rich Environments

1. Use parallel communication strategies at home and in school, e.g., speaking while signing (total communication approach), or alternating between languages based on context.
2. Incorporate visual aids, routines, and tactile supports to reinforce understanding.
3. Encourage meaningful interaction in both languages through play, daily routines, and social exchanges.

Use Professional Models and Fluent Language Partners

1. Provide access to fluent sign language users, such as deaf mentors or sign-fluent educators.
2. Ensure therapists and educators are trained in both spoken and signed language instruction.
3. Avoid relying on family members or interpreters alone to model language, especially if they are not proficient.

Incorporate Augmentative and Alternative Communication (AAC)

1. Introduce visual symbols or AAC devices as needed, to bridge gaps between spoken and signed communication.
2. Use AAC tools that support dual-language displays, where the child sees both a symbol and a signed/spoken equivalent.
3. AAC should support, not replace, natural language learning in both modalities (Geers & Nicholas, 2020).

Build Metalinguistic Awareness

1. Use age-appropriate strategies to help children understand when and why different languages are used.
2. Encourage code-switching where appropriate (e.g., using sign with deaf peers and speech with hearing individuals), but do not pressure the child to keep languages "separate" if that causes stress.

Collaborate Across Disciplines and Settings

1. Speech-language pathologists, audiologists, special educators, and sign language interpreters should work together to ensure continuity across settings.
2. IEP or IFSP teams should set language-specific goals (e.g., increasing expressive signs, improving verbal requests) and monitor progress in both languages (National Center for Learning Disabilities, 2023).
3. Family training and coaching are critical for generalizing skills beyond the clinic or classroom.

Respect and Support the Family's Language Goals

1. Some families may prioritize spoken language due to cultural or practical reasons; others may embrace deaf culture and sign language.
2. Professionals should guide families through informed decision-making, without bias toward one modality.
3. A family-centered approach ensures better engagement and long-term consistency in language use.

Table 4.4. key bilingual language-support strategies designed to strengthen communication development for children with Hearing Impairment

Strategy Area	*Key Actions*
Early and Consistent Exposure	Start both spoken and sign language early; use rich language input regularly in both modalities.
Language-Rich Environments	Use visuals, routines, and parallel communication (e.g., speak and sign together); encourage use in daily life.
Professional Language Models	Include deaf mentors, sign-fluent teachers, and trained therapists; avoid relying solely on non-fluent family members.
Use of AAC	Introduce AAC tools (e.g., symbol-based apps) that support both languages; AAC should enhance – not replace – natural language.
Metalinguistic Awareness	Teach when and why different languages are used; support code-switching without enforcing strict separation.
Interdisciplinary Collaboration	Coordinate goals among SLPs, audiologists, educators, and families; monitor progress in both languages via IEP/IFSP.
Family-Centered Approach	Respect cultural/language preferences; guide families without bias; support informed and consistent decisions.

Benefits of Bilingual Exposure in Dual Diagnosis

Research and practice indicate that children with ASD and Hearing Impairment can:

1. Learn and use both spoken and sign languages when appropriately supported.
2. Use different modalities for different purposes (e.g., signs for expression, speech for comprehension).
3. Show enhanced emotional regulation and behavioral adjustment when given tools for expressive communication.
4. Develop stronger social connections when communication is accessible and consistent.

Challenges and Considerations

1. Some children may favor one language over the other, this is natural and may vary over time.
2. Bilingual development may be uneven; one modality may be more developed depending on context or exposure (Marschark & Knoors, 2020).
3. Professionals must carefully assess language development in each modality, not assume progress in one reflects the other.

Supporting language acquisition in bilingual (spoken/sign) environments for children with dual diagnoses of ASD and hearing impairment requires an inclusive, flexible, and family-centered approach. With early exposure, consistent modeling, and collaboration among professionals, these children can develop meaningful communication in both modalities. Bilingual language development enhances not only linguistic competence but also social inclusion, emotional well-being, and educational success, making it a vital component of holistic intervention.

Three overarching modalities of communication, Speech, Sign Language, and Augmentative and Alternative Communication (AAC), which facilitate language development in people with ASD, hearing impairment (HI) or dual diagnosis. Each mode is a particular way of linguistic input and output that is directed by the sensory means, cognitive profiles and environmental exposures of the learner. Knowing their relative strengths and weaknesses can enable clinicians, educators, and families to choose and establish personalized multimodal communication systems that are inclusive, individualized and functionally relevant.

It is also verbal in nature and speech is the most popular form of communication. It relies on the integrity of audio system to input, process, and feedback on language. In children having a normal hearing ability, speech assists in incidental learning, phonological awareness and social interaction via prosody, tone, and rhythm. Nevertheless, spoken language might be limited to the impaired hearing or auditory processing condition of people with hearing impairment or speech processing deficits, despite the use of amplification devices such as hearing aids or cochlear implants. Echolalia, or pragmatic communication deficits may also complicate the speech development in children with ASD due to delayed language acquisition (Davidson & Quittner, 2020). Therefore, although speech is an important area of intervention, it cannot be the only method of communication among all learners, particularly when the sensory or neurodevelopmental profile restricts the auditory comprehension of the learner.

Sign language provides an entirely accessible, visual-manual language of communication that Deaf and Hard of Hearing (DHH) individuals cannot do

Table 4.5. Accessibility and input modes of speech, sign language, and AAC to guide effective multimodal communication planning

Aspect	*Speech*	*Sign Language*	*AAC*
Input Mode	Auditory	Visual	Visual/Touch
Accessibility	Needs hearing	Accessible to DHH	Universal
Example	Spoken words	ASL/PSL	PECS, tablet devices

without, and neurodiverse learners that better assimilate information using visual-spatial modalities find invaluable. Sign languages like American Sign Language (ASL) and Pakistan Sign Language (PSL) are grammatically closed systems that have a syntax, morphology, and cultural identity (Shield & Meier, 2020). Sign language is a tangible and visual expression of meaning, which helps children with ASD and HI in their understanding and expressive communication in situations where auditory communication is not possible or overwhelming. In addition, sign language has the potential of minimizing frustration and behavioral difficulties that occur in a breakdown of communication. Nonetheless, some difficulties can be experienced because of motor coordination problems, a deficiency in joint attention, or social reciprocity of the frequently experienced ASD. Being exposed to sign-rich environments in the early stages of life particularly in the family and school, which encourage the use of both the bimodal mode of communication, has a profound influence on language and cognitive performance. Therefore, sign language can be used as a means of communication, inclusion, identity, and cognition.

Augmentative and Alternative Communication (AAC) is a generalization of visual, tactile, and technological systems that are meant to be used to complement or substitute speech and sign. AAC consists of low-tech (Picture Exchange Communication System, PECS, and communication boards) and high-tech (speech-generating tablet devices, apps based on symbols, etc.) tools (Schlosser & Koul, 2021). In the case of children with dual diagnoses, experiencing multiple hindrance to auditory input, speech production, and pragmatic communication, AAC provides a universal, multimodal point of entry to expression. The fact that it has two senses: visual and tactile, enables it to have versatility in terms of sensory profiles, and its systematic symbol systems bring about understanding, predictability, and choice-making. As opposed to popular beliefs, the use of AAC does not hinder the development of speech or sign language; on the contrary, it can often contribute to both, improving the communicative purpose, learning new vocabulary, and cognitive involvement.

In the context of accessibility, speech is based on the processing of auditory files and therefore restricts to persons with severe hearing impairment. As a visual language, sign language can still be used by DHH communities, but receptive partners knowledgeable in sign would need to be involved. AAC on the other hand is universally accessible, flexible to auditory, visual, and cognitive differences and therefore works best in an inclusive classroom and family environment when there are more than two communication partners involved.

The examples in Table 4.1 – ASL/PSL of sign language, PECS or tablet-based system of AAC, spoken words of speech – demonstrate how each of the modes can be an independent system or supplementary to other systems in a multimodal communication structure. The combination of these approaches is becoming supported by evidence-based practice, which means that the individual can alternate between the modes based on the situation, comfort, and communicative objectives.

There is no universal best at communication mode, but the most effective one is the one that fits and is flexible. Speech provides a sense of social and linguistic immersion, sign language guarantees accessibility and visual cognition, and AAC fills the gaps in expressiveness and stimulates autonomy. In children with ASD and hearing impairment, auditory-verbal, visual-manual and technological multimodal communication plan is the best to enhance language development, emotional expression and involvement in various environments. This comparative model proposes equity in communication where all children, at whatever sensory or neurodevelopment profile, can access language in whatever form best represents their distinct manner of view and expression of the world.

Critical variables that play a significant role in the language development of children with hearing impairment (HI) both with co-occurring ASD or other neurodevelopmental variation. Although cochlear implants (CIs) provide astounding access to the auditory input, the successful language development is not entirely defined by the technological performance. Rather, it is mediated by an interaction between developmental timing, consistency of the therapeutic process, and family involvement, all of which mediate the ability of the child to map auditory access to meaningful communication.

One of the most definite predictors of linguistic and cognitive outcomes is Age at Implantation. Many longitudinal studies (e.g., Nicholas & Geers, 2017) show that the sooner implantation is done, preferably prior to the age of two, the better the speech perception, vocabulary acquisition, and syntactic development because the brain is most neuroplastic at early periods of auditory sensitivity. During this critical developmental period, the auditory cortex will tend to conform to sound as opposed to cross-modally reorganize when auditory stimulation is given (Kral & Sharma, 2012). Conversely, implantation can be delayed (particularly following long-term auditory deprivation) resulting in lower speech intelligibility and slower increase in comprehension because neural pathways have now developed to prioritarian visual/tactile stimuli. In the case of children with dual diagnoses, preimplantation should be accompanied by more specific communication interventions that consider both the needs of social-communicative and sensory regulation and make sure that the access of the ear can be translated into functional language.

Table 4.6. Key factors that significantly shape language and developmental outcomes in children with Hearing Impairment

Factor	*Influence on Development*
Age at Implantation	Earlier improves speech and comprehension.
Therapy Quality	Consistent sessions enhance outcomes.
Family Involvement	Home language exposure increases progress.

The second determinant of post-implant language outcome that is critical is Therapy Quality. It is not a panacea to restore sound with the help of the cochlear implant and guarantee understanding and speech success but rather sustained, qualitative auditory-verbal therapies and speech interventions that are necessary to train the auditory brain and linguistic generalization (Geers et al., 2019). Structured and regular therapy sessions assist children in distinguishing speech sounds, matching auditory information and meaning, as well as learning pragmatic language skills. Competent intervention should be multimodal, which involves listening, visuals, and learning in a context to support the understanding. In children with ASD and HI, the therapeutic models should be aimed at the combination of auditory training and social-communication scaffolding, with the emphasis on the production of words and intentionality, reciprocity, and emotional involvement. Home, clinic, and education continuity of services is critical in maintaining language gains in the long run.

The aspect of Family Involvement becomes one of the pillars of effective post-implant language development. Families offer the abundant linguistic environment that is needed to consolidate the therapeutic gains and converting auditory input into spontaneous communication. The studies continually emphasize that children whose caregivers involve themselves in day-to-day language stimulation, with the help of conversations, shared reading, play based interaction and responsive communication, experience more advancement in speech sensing, expansion of vocabulary and readiness to read literacy (DesJardin & Eisenberg, 2007). The family beliefs related to deafness; mode of communication and consistency of the intervention have a significant impact.

Parental learning about both auditory and neurodevelopmental aspects is critical in cases of dual diagnosis: the family will be faced with the need to balance auditory training with the comfort of the child and cognitive preparedness, which may involve the use of sign language or AAC resource along with the oral language. Not only does such an informed flexibility enhance language development, but also it decreases frustration and enhances emotion.

Altogether, the aspects listed in Table 4.2 point to the idea that cochlear implantation is not a single medical event but the initiator of the continuous developmental process that combines auditory, linguistic, and social experiences. The best results are achieved when environmental enrichment (family engagement and consistent therapy) coincides with biological opportunity (early implantation). In children with ASD and hearing impairment, success may not necessarily be determined by normative speech measures per se, but rather how much language, oral, signed or multimodal, allows a meaningful involvement, communication, and self-expression. Therefore, language development following cochlear implantation should be perceived as a complex process, a process which connects technology, neurodevelopment, and human relations in turning silence into knowledge.

Real-Life Situation: Sign and AAC Integration

Hamza was seven years old. He had ASD and profound hearing loss, with limited speech and poor signs. His therapist identified Pakistan Sign Language (PSL) and a picture-based AAC application, and, over time, Hamza started mixing picture requests and signs, e.g., eat and play. Educators experienced less meltdown as well as better classroom dynamics. The practical example provided on the application of sign language and AAC in enabling expressive communication to dual-diagnosis learners is realistic.

Summary

1 In dual diagnosis, communicating has to be a multimodal, flexible approach based on speech, sign and AAC systems.
2 Visual strategies and sign language provide concrete language models that are available to a large number of students.
3 Deficit in pragmatic and social language is magnified and requires direct, systematic instructions.
4 AAC systems do not pose any obstacle to speech or sign development as they bridge the communication gap.
5 Communication grow is maintained through family involvement and repetition in settings.

References

American Association on Intellectual and Developmental Disabilities. (2021). *Supports for transitioning youth with dual diagnoses*. https://www.aaidd.org.

Brady, N. C., Warren, Z., Fleming, K., Keller, J., & Sterling, L. (2021). Communication challenges in children with autism spectrum disorder who are deaf or hard of hearing. *Pediatrics*, 147(*Supplement* 2), e2020021982F. doi:10.1542/peds.2020-021982F.

Davidson, K. (2020). Bimodal bilingualism in deaf and hard-of-hearing children: Implications for cognitive and language development. *Journal of Deaf Studies and Deaf Education*, 25(3), 263–273. doi:10.1093/deafed/enz050.

Davidson, L. S., & Quittner, A. L. (2020). Pragmatic language development in children who are deaf or hard of hearing. *Journal of Speech, Language, and Hearing Research*, 63(7), 2131–2145. doi:10.1044/2020_JSLHR-19-00234.

Deaf Child Worldwide. (2021). *Social communication and access to language for deaf children globally*. https://www.deafchildworldwide.info.

Geers, A. E., Moog, J. S., Biedenstein, J., Nicholas , J. G., & Sedey, A. L. (2019). Early auditory experience and language development in children who are deaf or hard of hearing: Findings from a prospective longitudinal study. *Ear and Hearing*, 40(1), 20–38. doi:10.1097/AUD.0000000000000610.

Geers, A. E., & Nicholas, J. G. (2020). Language and spoken communication outcomes for children with cochlear implants. *Pediatrics*, 146(Supplement 3), S262–S270. doi:10.1542/peds.2020-0242E.

Giangreco, M. F. (2021). *Inclusive education for students with significant communication needs: Collaboration, support, and access*. Brookes Publishing.

Glickman, N. S., & Hall, W. C. (2021). *Language deprivation and deaf mental health*. Routledge.

Harris, M. S., Kronenberger, W. G., Gao, S., Hoen, H. M., Miyamoto, R. T., & Pisoni, D. B. (2021). Executive functioning in children with cochlear implants. *Ear and Hearing*, 42(1), 72–86. doi:10.1097/AUD.0000000000000905.

Kral, A., & Sharma, A. (2012). Developmental neuroplasticity after cochlear implantation. *Trends in Neurosciences*, 35(2), 111–122. doi:10.1016/j.tins.2011.09.004.

Marschark, M., & Knoors, H. (2020). Bilingual development in deaf children. In H. Knoors & M. Marschark (Eds.), *Educating deaf learners: Research, practice, and policy* (pp. 29–51). Oxford University Press.

Nicholas, J. G., & Geers, A. E. (2017). Early intervention and language outcomes in children with cochlear implants. *Ear and Hearing*, 39(6), 112–123. doi:10.1097/AUD.0000000000000563.

Schlosser, R. W., & Koul, R. (2021). *Augmentative and alternative communication: Assessment and intervention strategies*. Plural Publishing.

Shield, A., & Meier, R. P. (2020). Sign language acquisition in children with autism spectrum disorder and hearing loss. *Journal of Deaf Studies and Deaf Education*, 25 (2), 123–135. doi:10.1093/deafed/enz052.

Thiemann-Bourque, K., & Brady, N. (2021). Peer-mediated interventions to support social communication in children with autism spectrum disorder. *Topics in Early Childhood Special Education*, 41(2), 70–81. doi:10.1177/0271121420912987.

Chapter 5

Educational and Behavioral Interventions

Evidence-based Practices for Learners with ASD and hearing impairment

Learners with co-occurring Autism Spectrum Disorder (ASD) and hearing impairment represent a highly diverse and complex population. Their educational and therapeutic needs span across communication, behavior, social interaction, and sensory processing. To ensure meaningful progress, it is essential to use evidence-based practices (EBPs), interventions that are supported by rigorous research, adapted to the dual needs of the learner, and implemented with fidelity (Odom et al., 2021; National Autism Center, 2020; Hampton & Kaiser, 2020).

While research specifically targeting the dual diagnosis population remains limited, a growing body of literature supports the adaptation of well-established EBPs for ASD and hearing loss when used in integrated, individualized, and multimodal formats.

Structured Teaching (TEACCH Approach)

The TEACCH (Treatment and Education of Autistic and Communication-Handicapped Children) approach emphasizes structure, routine, and visual supports, elements that benefit both children with ASD and those with hearing loss. Key strategies include:

1 Visual schedules, work systems, and environmental organization.
2 Task structuring using visual or tactile prompts.
3 Predictable routines to reduce anxiety and improve engagement.

For DHH learners, instructions, and supports must be accessible through sign language, visual cues, or AAC, depending on the child's needs.

DOI: 10.4324/9781003750611-5

Applied Behavior Analysis (ABA) with Communication Supports

ABA is a well-researched, widely used framework for teaching functional skills to learners with ASD. When adapted for DHH children, ABA remains effective (Burke & Hodapp, 2020), particularly when focusing on:

1 Functional communication training (FCT).
2 Positive reinforcement for social behaviors and language use.
3 Discrete trial training (DTT) using visual or signed prompts.

Communication modes should be individualized (spoken, signed, AAC), and therapists must be fluent in or have access to professionals fluent in the child's communication language.

Visual Supports and AAC

Visual supports are core components of many EBPs and are highly effective for learners with ASD and hearing loss due to their visual learning strengths. Common visual strategies include:

1 Picture Exchange Communication System (PECS).
2 Visual schedules and cue cards.
3 Social stories with visual narratives.
4 Speech-generating devices (SGDs) or symbol-based AAC apps.

Research shows that AAC use can increase expressive language, reduce behavioral frustration, and support social interactions, especially in minimally verbal learners.

Social Skills Training and Peer-Mediated Instruction

Children with ASD and hearing impairment often have limited opportunities for social learning. Structured social skills programs, adapted to the child's communication mode, can teach (Thiemann-Bourque & Brady, 2021):

1 Turn-taking.
2 Joint attention.
3 Conversation initiation and maintenance.

Peer-mediated interventions, where typically developing peers are trained to model and reinforce social behaviors, are effective, especially when combined with visual prompts or sign language (Thiemann-Bourque & Brady, 2021).

Total Communication Approach

The Total Communication (TC) philosophy promotes the simultaneous use of multiple communication modes, spoken language, sign language, gestures, pictures, and written words, based on the child's individual strengths and preferences.

Research supports TC for children with hearing loss and, when used with learners on the autism spectrum, it allows flexibility and reduces communication barriers. TC is most effective when:

1. Implemented consistently across home, school, and therapy.
2. Tailored to cognitive and sensory profiles.
3. Supported by professionals trained in bimodal language instruction.

Parent-Mediated Interventions

Parents are central to the success of any EBP. Parent-mediated interventions, such as Pivotal Response Treatment (PRT) and Hanen's "More Than Words", have demonstrated positive outcomes in both communication and behavior (Zaidman-Zait & Curle, 2020).

When adapted for families of children with hearing loss:

1. Training includes modeling signed or AAC-based communication.
2. Emphasis is placed on creating language-rich, visually accessible interactions.
3. Coaching and video feedback improve parental responsiveness and child engagement.

Sensory Integration Strategies

Learners with ASD often experience sensory processing difficulties, and hearing impairment can further complicate auditory, tactile, and vestibular integration. Occupational therapy (OT) strategies rooted in Ayres Sensory Integration (ASI) can support:

1. Regulation.
2. Attention.
3. Functional participation.

These interventions are most effective when sensory activities are:

1. Visually guided.
2. Aligned with the child's sensory profile.
3. Integrated into daily routines.

Early Intervention and Interdisciplinary Collaboration

Early intervention, ideally before the age of three, is critical for optimizing language, cognitive, and social development (Hampton & Kaiser, 2020). Successful EBPs in early childhood settings include:

1 Joint attention training.
2 Play-based interventions.
3 Developmental social-pragmatic (DSP) approaches.

Intervention must be delivered through interdisciplinary collaboration involving:

1 Audiologists.
2 Speech-language pathologists.
3 Special educators.
4 Occupational therapists.
5 Behavior specialists.
6 Family members.

Conclusion

Evidence-based practices for learners with ASD and hearing impairment must be individualized, multimodal, and collaborative. While most EBPs were originally designed for one population, thoughtful adaptation and interdisciplinary implementation make them effective for children with dual diagnoses (Odom et al., 2021). By combining the principles of structured teaching, visual communication, behavioral reinforcement, and family involvement, professionals can create inclusive, accessible learning environments that promote communication, independence, and social connection (Cekaite & Ekström, 2022).

Structured Teaching, Visual Supports, and Applied Behavior Analysis (ABA) Adaptations

For learners with dual diagnoses of ASD and hearing impairment, evidence-based interventions must be thoughtfully adapted to address communication challenges, sensory sensitivities, and unique learning profiles. Three widely used and effective approaches – structured teaching, visual supports, and Applied Behavior Analysis (ABA) – offer substantial benefits when modified to accommodate the needs of this diverse population. These interventions leverage the child's strengths in visual processing, routine-based learning, and reinforcement-based instruction, making them highly relevant in inclusive and specialized educational settings (Odom et al., 2021; Hampton & Kaiser, 2020).

Structured Teaching

Structured teaching, originally developed through the TEACCH (Treatment and Education of Autistic and Communication-handicapped Children) program, provides an environment that emphasizes predictability, routine, and visual organization, all essential for learners with ASD and hearing impairment.

Core Components and Benefits

1. Physical structure: Clearly defined spaces for specific activities (e.g., work area, play area) help reduce distractions and support task engagement.
2. Visual schedules: Sequential visual representations of daily routines reduce anxiety and support transition management, especially important for children who cannot rely on verbal prompts (American Association on Intellectual and Developmental Disabilities, 2021).
3. Work systems: Step-by-step task breakdowns using pictures, symbols, or objects assist learners in understanding task expectations and promoting independence.

Adaptations for Dual Diagnosis

1. Incorporate signed instructions, visual gestures, or AAC symbols in all routines.
2. Ensure environments are visually accessible, well-lit, low-clutter, and optimized for eye-level displays.
3. Pair real objects or tactile cues with visuals for learners with limited symbolic understanding.

Visual Supports

Visual supports are essential tools for enhancing comprehension, expression, and emotional regulation in learners who struggle with auditory or verbal language. These supports benefit both autistic learners and those who are Deaf or Hard of Hearing (DHH), as they rely on visual strengths rather than auditory processing.

Examples of Visual Supports

1. Visual schedules (e.g., first-then boards, daily timelines).
2. Choice boards and communication cards.
3. Emotion thermometers, behavior expectation charts, and rule posters.
4. Social stories with picture-based narratives for teaching routines and social norms.

Adaptations for Learners with ASD and hearing impairment

1 Use sign language-integrated visuals, such as symbols paired with sign cues or fingerspelling images.
2 Provide consistent visual labeling in classrooms and homes for object recognition and vocabulary building.
3 For nonreaders, employ photo-based supports or tactile symbols.
4 Reinforce visuals with gesture, modeling, and consistent routines across environments.

Applied Behavior Analysis (ABA) Adaptations

Applied Behavior Analysis (ABA) is a highly structured, data-driven approach that uses positive reinforcement to teach new skills and reduce problematic behaviors. ABA has shown strong efficacy for individuals with ASD and is increasingly adapted for use with children who have hearing impairment.

Core ABA Strategies

1 Discrete Trial Training (DTT): Repetitive, structured teaching trials that include a prompt, response, and reinforcement.
2 Natural Environment Teaching (NET): Instruction embedded in daily routines and play.
3 Functional Communication Training (FCT): Teaching communication as a replacement for challenging behavior.

Adaptations for Dual Diagnosis

1 Replace or supplement verbal prompts with visual, signed, or tactile prompts.
2 Ensure therapists are fluent in the child's primary communication mode (sign language, AAC, etc.).
3 Modify reinforcers to align with visual or sensory preferences (e.g., visual spinning toys, light-up rewards).
4 Use video modeling and task analysis to break down complex behaviors into visual sequences.
5 Collect data on both communication modality uses and behavioral progress to assess effectiveness.

ABA for learners with hearing impairment must go beyond spoken-language-based expectations and embrace multimodal communication systems, using what is most effective and accessible for each child.

Integration Across Approaches

The synergy of structured teaching, visual supports, and ABA creates an integrated learning environment where:

1 Predictability and visual access increase confidence and independence.
2 Motivation and reinforcement drive skill acquisition.
3 Communication systems are honored and expanded, whether through sign, AAC, or visual cues.

Professionals should collaborate to implement these strategies across home, school, and therapeutic settings, ensuring consistency, generalization, and progress monitoring.

Conclusion

Structured teaching, visual supports, and ABA, when adapted thoughtfully, form a powerful framework for addressing the complex needs of learners with ASD and hearing impairment. These strategies respect the learners' sensory and communicative strengths while systematically building foundational skills for independence, social engagement, and academic success. By prioritizing visual accessibility, functional communication, and individualized reinforcement, educators and therapists can create inclusive and effective intervention environments that empower each child to thrive.

Classroom Accommodations and Environmental Modifications

Creating an inclusive and supportive classroom environment is essential for learners with dual diagnoses of Autism Spectrum Disorder (ASD) and hearing impairment. These students face multifaceted challenges in areas such as communication, sensory regulation, attention, and social interaction. Therefore, effective classroom accommodations and environmental modifications must address both the sensory and neurodevelopmental profiles of these learners, enabling access to the curriculum, fostering independence, and promoting participation.

Acoustic and Visual Accessibility

Acoustic Modifications

While students with hearing impairment rely on assistive listening devices, optimal acoustic conditions are critical. Poor classroom acoustics can compromise both amplified auditory input and the ability to focus.

- Install sound-field amplification systems or personal FM/DM systems.
- Use carpeting, acoustic panels, or ceiling tiles to reduce echo and background noise.
- Seat the student away from noisy areas, such as windows, fans, or hallways.

Visual Accessibility

Since visual input is a primary source of information for DHH and ASD learners:

- Ensure clear sight lines to the teacher, interpreter, visual aids, and peers.
- Use well-lit classrooms without glare or flickering lights.
- Provide visual supports such as captioned videos, picture instructions, and illustrated materials.

Communication Accommodations

Children with dual diagnoses may use spoken language, sign language, AAC, or a combination. The classroom must accommodate these modes consistently.

1. Provide trained sign language interpreters or communication facilitators when needed.
2. Allow the use of speech-generating devices, picture exchange systems (PECS), or visual communication boards.
3. Incorporate total communication approaches, pairing speech with signs or symbols to support comprehension.
4. Teachers and peers should be trained in basic communication strategies relevant to the child's needs (e.g., using signs, slowing speech, and maintaining eye contact).

Physical Layout and Classroom Design

A well-structured physical environment supports focus, reduces anxiety, and enhances independence.

1. Clearly define learning areas (e.g., group work, reading corner, sensory zone) using furniture, visual markers, or colored rugs.
2. Minimize visual clutter to reduce distraction.
3. Use visual schedules, task boards, and "first-then" charts to structure activities and transitions.
4. Ensure seating arrangements allow for peer interaction, interpreter access, and teacher visibility.

Sensory-Friendly Modifications

Both ASD and hearing loss can affect sensory regulation. Some students may be hypersensitive to certain inputs, while others may seek additional stimulation.

1. Create a quiet corner or sensory break area where the student can self-regulate.
2. Offer access to noise-reducing headphones, fidget tools, or weighted items as needed.
3. Avoid harsh lighting, strong smells (e.g., from cleaning products), or crowded layouts that can overwhelm sensory systems.
4. Allow movement breaks or alternate seating options (e.g., wiggle cushions, standing desks).

Instructional and Curriculum Adaptations

To promote engagement and understanding, adapt the curriculum to be multisensory, visual, and hands-on.

1. Provide visual instructions and step-by-step demonstrations alongside verbal explanations.
2. Break tasks into manageable chunks with clear start and finish cues.
3. Use concrete materials and real-life contexts to enhance comprehension.
4. Allow extra processing time and provide visual cues during group discussions or transitions.
5. Use peer support or buddy systems to model appropriate behavior and facilitate communication.

Behavioral and Social Support Accommodations

ASD is often associated with behavioral challenges and social communication difficulties, which may be heightened in unfamiliar or unpredictable environments (Clark & Adams, 2023).

1. Implement positive behavior support plans (PBSPs) tailored to individual triggers and motivators.
2. Use visual behavior charts and token systems to reinforce expected behavior.
3. Teach explicit social skills using role-play, video modeling, and social stories.
4. Create predictable routines with visual cues and transitional warnings to reduce anxiety.

Collaboration with Specialists and Families

Effective accommodations require collaboration between general educators, special educators, therapists, and families.

1 Include input from audiologists, speech-language pathologists, occupational therapists, and behavior specialists in classroom planning.
2 Maintain consistent communication with families to reinforce strategies at home.
3 Incorporate Individualized Education Plan (IEP) or Individualized Learning Plan (ILP) goals into daily instruction (National Center for Learning Disabilities, 2023).

Table 5.1. Essential classroom modifications that support accessibility, communication, sensory needs, instruction, and collaboration for learners with diverse abilities

Area	*Key Modifications*
Acoustic and Visual Accessibility	Use FM/DM systems or sound-field amplification. Reduce noise with carpets and acoustic panels. Ensure clear sight lines and good lighting. Use captioned videos and visual aids.
Communication Accommodations	Provide sign language interpreters or facilitators. Support AAC tools like PECS or SGDs. Use total communication (speech + signs). Train teachers/peers in communication strategies.
Physical Layout and Classroom Design	Define areas using visual markers. Minimize clutter and distractions. Use visual schedules and task boards. Arrange seating for visibility and interaction.
Sensory-Friendly Modifications	Create quiet/sensory spaces. Provide noise-cancelling headphones or sensory tools. Avoid harsh lighting and strong smells. Allow movement breaks and flexible seating.
Instructional and Curriculum Adaptations	Use visual and hands-on materials. Break tasks into clear steps. Offer extra time and visual cues. Use peer support or buddy systems.
Behavioral and Social Supports	Implement PBSPs for individual needs. Use behavior charts and reinforcement systems. Teach social skills with modeling and stories. Maintain predictable routines with visual cues.
Collaboration with Specialists and Families	Involve therapists and special educators in planning. Communicate regularly with families. Align teaching with IEP/ILP goals.

Conclusion

Learners with ASD and hearing impairment thrive in classrooms that are structured, visually accessible, and sensory-aware, where communication is intentional and inclusive, and where teachers are flexible, responsive, and collaborative. By making thoughtful accommodations and modifications, educators not only improve access to learning but also promote engagement, autonomy, and social belonging for every learner.

Collaborating with Families in Intervention Planning

Family collaboration is a cornerstone of effective intervention for children with ASD and hearing impairment. These dual diagnoses present complex communication, behavioral, and sensory challenges that affect not only the child but the entire family system. Meaningful, respectful collaboration with families ensures that interventions are individualized, culturally sensitive, and consistent across settings, ultimately leading to better developmental, social, and educational outcomes (Hampton & Kaiser, 2020).

Importance of Family Collaboration

Families are the primary advocates, caregivers, and language models for their children. They hold deep knowledge of their child's history, preferences, routines, and communication styles. In dual diagnosis cases, collaboration is especially vital because:

1. Families must often navigate multiple systems, healthcare, audiology, special education, and disability services.
2. Intervention success depends on consistency across home and school.
3. Parents may be managing emotional stress, decision-making pressures, and learning multiple communication systems (e.g., sign language, AAC, therapy techniques).

When professionals partner with families rather than direct them, the result is a more empowered, informed, and engaged support system around the child.

Principles of Effective Family Collaboration

Respect and Empathy

1. Acknowledge the family's unique experiences, cultural background, and emotional journey.
2. Show empathy toward challenges such as grief, uncertainty, or past negative experiences with service systems.

Shared Decision-Making

1 Involve families in goal-setting, therapy planning, and instructional strategies.
2 Use clear, jargon-free language when explaining assessments, progress, and interventions.
3 Validate parents' insights and preferences regarding communication mode, priorities, and daily routines.

Cultural and Linguistic Sensitivity

1 Recognize and honor the family's linguistic preferences, whether spoken language, sign language, or bilingual communication.
2 Adapt materials and interventions to fit the cultural values and practices of the family.
3 Provide interpreters or bilingual support staff when needed to ensure full understanding and participation.

Strategies for Involving Families in Intervention Planning

Regular Communication

1 Maintain ongoing communication through parent–teacher logs, phone calls, video messages, or home visits.
2 Use visual aids, translated materials, or demonstration videos to share strategies.
3 Set regular meetings to review progress, challenges, and adjustments to intervention plans.

Parent Training and Coaching

1 Offer training sessions on:
2 Sign language or AAC use.
3 Behavioral strategies (e.g., prompting, reinforcement).
4 Creating language-rich environments at home.
5 Provide modeling, feedback, and hands-on practice during sessions.
6 Use video modeling and video feedback to support parents in applying strategies confidently.

Home-Based Suppors Activities

1 Design home programs with achievable, meaningful goals (e.g., increasing turn-taking during meals, using signs for basic requests).
2 Include visual schedules or routines that mirror those used at school or therapy.

3 Ensure activities are flexible and adapted to family resources and time constraints.

Empowerment through Information

1 Share current information about ASD, hearing loss, bilingual development, and intervention options.
2 Encourage families to ask questions, attend workshops, and join support networks.
3 Support families in understanding IEP/IFSP processes and advocating for their child's needs.

Benefits of Family–Professional Collaboration

Collaborative intervention planning leads to:

1 Stronger generalization of skills across environments.
2 Earlier identification of issues or regression.
3 Increased family confidence and satisfaction.
4 Improved long-term outcomes in communication, behavior, and emotional well-being.

Children benefit most when home and school environments work together, reinforcing the same expectations and celebrating the same successes. Collaborating with families is not a supplementary component of intervention; it is an essential and ethical practice, particularly for children with ASD and hearing impairment. By building trusting partnerships, professionals can co-create interventions that are personalized, consistent, and sustainable, ultimately supporting the child's development in ways that are culturally appropriate, functionally relevant, and emotionally supportive. Family centered intervention planning leads not only to better outcomes for the child, but also to empowered, resilient families capable of advocating for and nurturing their child's potential (Kyzar & Turnbull, 2021).

Case Study 1:Structured Teaching of a Multisensory Classroom (TEACCH Framework)

Context

One such student at a mainstream inclusive school was a nine-year-old student called Sana who has ASD and moderate hearing impairment and was unable to transition in and out of classroom and complete tasks.

Intervention

Her teacher adopted the TEACCH model, making it visually and kinesthetically adaptable. The classroom was broken into distinct areas of activity (Reading Corner, Writing Desk, Sensory Area). There were visual instructions with colors and PSL (Pakistan Sign Language) symbols at each station.

Outcome

Sana also improved her on-task behavior by 60% and her anxiety during transitions had reduced after four weeks. She started to make the communication first with the help of signs.

Practical Insight

Visual schedules and routines allow dual-diagnosis students to be focused and self-sufficient and minimize sensory overload and aggressive behavior (Pfeiffer & Milligan, 2023).

Case Study 2: Preparing ABA to Meet Dual Diagnosis

Context

Ahmed is a seven-year-old boy with ASD; he is severely bilaterally deaf and also displayed repetitive tapping and withdrawal of group play.

Intervention

Applied Behavior Analysis (ABA) principles were modified to his requirements by a behavior analyst and special educator together. They substituted verbal prompts with the use of signed and pictorial cues, token rewards, and visual feedback charts. Preferred sensory activities (sand play and water beads) were also used as reinforcement.

Outcome

Within two months, Ahmed's the repetitive tapping had decreased by 40% in addition to him now taking part in peer circle-time through sign gestures.

Practical Insight

Tangible reinforcement and visual–behavioral prompting assist in the structure of ABA and the needs of the child in relation to his or her sensory and linguistic accessibility.

Case Study 3: Collaboration in the Family, and the Total Communication Approach

Context

Maria was 10 years old. She wore a cochlear implant and possessed rather typical features of ASD in her pragmatic language. Her parents would only talk and speak at home, which would frustrate her and cause her to become more aggressive.

Intervention

A Total Communication plan was created consisting of speech and PSL, as well as visual picture cues. The parents were trained on the combination of spoken words and signs on a weekly basis, whereas the teachers engaged in uniform multimodal approaches.

Outcome

After a period of10 weeks, Maria was able to independently communicate in sign and speech both at home and school. The number of her behavioral incidences reduced significantly, and she became socially more reciprocal.

Practical Insight

The consistency of communication between the family members enhances the generalization and the emotional security. Multimodal integration enables verbal and non-verbal learning to be integrated and learner to express themselves fully.

Practical Illustrations and Case Studies

The case studies that follow are an illustration of how educational and behavioral interventions can be modified to accommodate children with Autism Spectrum Disorder and hearing impairment. These are practical examples of classroom, therapeutic and home based applications of structured teaching, behavioral adaptation and family engagement strategies.

This provides a summary of three most popular known evidence-based intervention models – Applied Behavior Analysis (ABA) Adaptations; TEACCH; and Functional Communication Training (FCT) – that have proved effective in helping individuals with ASD, HI, and dual diagnosis. Although each of these methods has a unique theoretical orientation and application, all of them have a common purpose, which is to encourage adaptive behavior, increase the ability to communicate, and engage in meaningful activities both

Table 5.2. Key intervention approaches, their primary focus areas, and simple practical examples used with learners

Approach	*Focus Area*	*Example*
ABA Adaptations	Behavior modification	Visual cues + reinforcement
TEACCH	Structured teaching	Visual schedules
FCT	Communication replacement	Request-based intervention

in the educational and social settings. Both frameworks have been modified to fit the individual sensory and communicative profiles of the children with both neurodevelopmental and auditory dissimilarities.

ABA Adaptations are still considered to be basic in the behavioral treatment of ASD, believed to focus on the systematic application of principles of reinforcement to form desirable forms of behavior and to diminish other forms of behavior (Cooper, Heron, & Heward, 2020). In the dual-diagnostic contexts, though, the conventional ABA procedures should be sensory and communication-receptive. Modifications involve incorporation of visual aids and sign support together with gestures as an alternative to verbal instructions in case of limited access to auditory instructions. The reinforcement strategies are rendered multimodal, i.e. visual tokens, tactile feedback, or sign-based praise are accompanied by traditional verbal reinforcement.

In the case of Deaf or Hard of Hearing (DHH) children, ABA involves more visual interaction and organized transitions with routine elements that help them lessen anxiety and develop a better understanding. Notably, ABA among this group takes the form of a compliance-based model which is turned into a communication-based model. The emphasis is not necessarily on the minimization of problem behavior; rather, teaching of functional and self-owned alternatives that are congruent with communication skills and sensory sensibilities of the individual.

The TEACCH (Treatment and Education of Autistic and Communication-Handicapped Children) method offers a systematic teaching system that takes advantage of organizing visually, predictability of the environment, and personal instruction (Mesibov & Shea, 2010). Based on the ideas of cognitive-behavioral learning, TEACCH builds on the visual profiles that are usually displayed by autistic and DHH students. This can be achieved through visual schedules, well-structured work systems, and spatial physical arrangement, which would improve autonomy and minimise dependency on verbal directives. To students who have a co-occurring diagnosis, TEACCH establishes a very open learning space to eliminate sensory overload and encourage interest in routine and clarity. The scaffolding visual symbols or sign-based labels are based on consistent visual symbols used by educators and therapists to help learners have a clear understanding of expectations and transitions throughout the day. The formal quality of TEACCH is not only useful in regulation of behavior but also in developing self-determination and self-confidence, which are essential to the children who are moving through a complicated world of both sensory and communication experiences.

Functional Communication Training (FCT) is a type of behavioral therapy that focuses on communication. It aims to remove undesired actions and replace them with more accountable communicative ones (Durand & Moskowitz, 2016), and works particularly in children with ASD and hearing impairment in which the behavioral outbursts are frequently due to frustration in communication. FCT is based on finding the purpose of problematic behaviors (e.g., wanting to escape a task, attaining attention, asking to take a break) and teaching an equivalent communicative response (e.g., a sign, gesture, symbol, or AAC expression) in a systematic manner so that the behavior can lead to the same outcome. As an example, a child with self-injury to prevent overstimulation will be trained to sign or use an AAC symbol to ask to take a sensory break.

This intervention needs to be visually anchored in DHH populations and with regular sign or symbol systems to provide clarity. With the alignment of the behavioral management approach with the communication empowerment approach, FCT represents the turn toward the positive, person-centered, and autonomy-supportive approaches to intervention.

Table 5.2 highlights that implementing proper educational and behavioral programs with individuals with dual diagnoses requires an integrated approach, adaptation, and sensitivity to context. All of the methods– ABA, TEACCH, and FCT – provide a framework that could be adjusted to the respect of sensory access, communication modality, and individual strengths. Together as a part of an interdisciplinary education strategy, these evidence-based interventions not only ensure the regulation of behavior but also encourage language development, emotional mood, and inclusion. This shift towards multimodal flexible neurodiversity-affirming practices as an intervention science is a major development in the study of intervention science that has made it more a matter of communication than behaviour management, more a matter of structure than empowerment and more a matter of therapy than human connection.

Table 5.3. **Strategies strengthening home–school collaboration through training, communication, and shared planning**

Strategy	*Description*
Parent Training	Educate parents on consistent methods.
Home–School Logs	Daily communication between teachers and families.
Collaborative IEPs	Shared goal-setting and progress review.

The importance of family–school collaboration as the core of maximizing educational, communicative, and behavioral outcome in children with ASD, hearing impairment (HI), or dual diagnosis is shown in Table 5.3. The school–home communication is a two-way support system since the communication between the school and home is regular, decisions are joint, and respect is taken into consideration so that the interventions are consistent between settings. Considering that children with dual diagnoses need to negotiate multifaceted learning, sensory, and communication settings, the integration of educators, therapists, and families is not a matter of choice but a prerequisite to development and eventual inclusion.

Parent training is the foundation of effective collaboration. Evidence-based knowledge and practical strategies to empower the parents will guarantee continuity between professional interventions and home-based reinforcement in the parents (Brookman-Frazee et al., 2006). Parent training refers to structured courses that teach the caregivers the concept of behavioral change, communication improvement, and sensory control to allow them to use the same style throughout the routine. Indicatively, the parents can be taught to utilize visual aids, sign-based signals, or reinforcement programs that are in tandem with the classroom practices. In the case of dual diagnosis, such training should also include understanding hearing technologies (hearing aids, cochlear implants) and communication modalities (speech, sign, AAC) to enable families to continue exposure to language and auditory learning at home. It has always been found that a child whose parents know the rationale of the intervention and actively engage in its implementation has higher behavioral stability, faster language acquisition, and better generalization of acquired skills in different environments (Oono, Honey, & McConachie, 2013).

Home–School logs offer an ordered and approachable way of everyday communication between families, therapists, and teachers. These records, whether written, electronic, or pictorial, record child performance and behavior, therapy objectives, and home activity on a daily basis. Such communication tools are fundamental to continuity across contexts in case the students with ASD and HI have a problem with expressing their experiences verbally. Home–School logs enable parents to practice classroom skills at home and also give the teacher feedback about the sleep, health, or behavior patterns of the child at home that can affect classroom operation. These logs may include visual symbols or sign-based summaries to allow less literate or hearing family members to the dual-diagnosis program. Home-school communication through consistent use fosters trust, openness, and mutual responsibility. Both settings are maintained in tandem with the developmental process of the child.

The Collaborative Individualized Education Programs (IEP) is the institutional form of family–school cooperation. In collaborative IEPs, educators, parents, audiologists, psychologists, and speech-language pathologists have shared goal-setting, frequent reviews of progress, and co-decision-making. This is a participatory model that ensures the educational objectives are not solely based on professional evaluations, but also on family concerns, cultural orientations, and communication orientations (Turnbull et al., 2021). Collaborative IEPs can be used with children with ASD and HI, combining dual-focus goals, relating to both auditory–verbal and social-communication development and clarifying accommodations like interpreters, captioning, visual aids, or sensory aids. Co-development and reviewing of IEPs are also beneficial in terms of developing stronger parental advocacy and agency, where parents are viewed not as passive recipients of professional guidance. This feeling of collaboration promotes continuity, inspiration, and empowerment throughout the child developmental ecosystem.

Together, Table 5.3 highlights that effective education of neurodiverse and sensory-diverse students cannot be achieved only in the context of expert-developed interventions but through the long-term and two-way cooperation of all stakeholders. The competence is developed in parent training, the communication is maintained with home-school logs, and shared responsibility is institutionalized through collaborative IEPs. Once these strategies are inculcated in the culture of the school, the outcome will be an inclusive, trust-based system in which family and teachers partner to help the child develop, gain independence, and become resilient. Simply, family–school partnership changes education as a location of education into an alternate, where learning extends beyond classrooms and progress is sustained through collective commitment.

Real-world Situation: Independence Visual Timetable

Nadia is a nine-year-old student with ASD and cochlear implants who tended to resist subject shifts. Her special teacher presented a visual program in the form of color-coded icons and sign indicators of day-to-day activities. In several weeks, Nadia adhered to routines on her own and she did not need verbal prompts as much. Her parents also recreated the system at home, which minimized the stress morning. As presented in the case, organized instruction and visual schemes advance self-regulation and predictability in general classrooms.

Summary

1 ASD and hearing-loss strategies should be incorporated into evidence-based practices in the inclusive educational environments.
2 Classroom participation and predictability is enhanced through the use of structured teaching, visual aids, and ABA adaptations.
3 Complete communication and environments that are controlled by senses lessens frustration and promotes learning.
4 Skill generalization is also strengthened by family input and home–school partnership.
5 Continued training of the professionals provides fidelity and sensitivity to dual needs.

References

American Association on Intellectual and Developmental Disabilities. (2021). *Supports for transitioning youth with dual diagnoses.* https://www.aaidd.org.

Brookman-Frazee, L., Stahmer, A., Baker-Ericzén, M. J., & Tsai, K. (2006). Parenting interventions for children with autism spectrum and disruptive behavior disorders: Opportunities for cross-fertilization. *Clinical Child and Family Psychology Review*, 9 (3–4),181–200. doi:10.1007/s10567-006-0010-4.

Burke, M. M., & Hodapp, R. M. (2020). *Developmental disabilities: Etiology, assessment, and intervention.* Springer.

Cekaite, A., & Ekström, A. (2022). *Child-directed interactions and multimodal communication in special education settings. Journal of Communication Disorders, 96,* 106188. doi:10.1016/j.jcomdis.2022.106188.

Clark, M. L., & Adams, R. D. (2023). Behavioral and social interventions for children with autism: Evidence-based classroom strategies. *Journal of Autism and Developmental Practice*, 12 (3), 145–160.

Cooper, J. O., Heron, T. E., & Heward, W. L. (2020). *Applied behavior analysis* (3rd edn.). Pearson.

Durand, V. M., & Moskowitz, L. J. (2016). Functional communication training: Thirty years of treating challenging behavior. *Topics in Early Childhood Special Education*, 36 (1), 28–35. doi:10.1177/0271121415626131.

Hampton, L. H., & Kaiser, A. P. (2020). Intervention effects on spoken-language outcomes for children with autism: A systematic review and meta-analysis. *Journal of Speech, Language, and Hearing Research*, 63 (11), 3785–3800. doi:10.1044/2020_JSLHR-20-00109.

Kyzar, K. B., & Turnbull, A. P. (2021). Family–professional partnerships and family-centered practices: A foundational guide for supporting families. *Infants & Young Children*, 34 (1), 3–17. doi:10.1097/IYC.0000000000000170.

Mesibov, G. B., & Shea, V. (2010). The TEACCH program in the era of evidence-based practice. *Journal of Autism and Developmental Disorders*, 40(5), 570–579. doi:10.1007/s10803-009-0901-6.

National Autism Center. (2020). *National standards project: Evidence-based practices for autism spectrum disorder (Phase 3).* Randolph, MA: National Autism Center at May Institute.

National Center for Learning Disabilities. (2023). *Individualized learning plans: Best practices for inclusive classrooms.* https://www.ncld.org.

Odom, S. L., Hall, L. J., Suhrheinrich, J., & Hume, K. (2021). Evidence-based practices for children and youth with autism: A comprehensive review. *Autism Research and Practice*, 4 (1), 1–16.

Oono, I. P., Honey, E. J., & McConachie, H. (2013). Parent-mediated early intervention for young children with autism spectrum disorders (ASD). *Cochrane Database of Systematic Reviews, 2013*(4), Article CD009774. doi:10.1002/14651858.CD009774.pub2.

Pfeiffer, B., & Milligan, S. (2023). Sensory and behavioral supports in autism and hearing impairment: Classroom implications of multimodal interventions. *American Journal of Occupational Therapy*, 77 (1), 1–12. doi:10.5014/ajot.2023.XXXXXX.

Thiemann-Bourque, K., & Brady, N. (2021). Social communication interventions for children with complex communication needs: Enhancing peer interactions. *American*

Journal of Speech-Language Pathology, 30 (1), 211–225. doi:10.1044/2020_AJSLP-20-00012.

Turnbull, A. P., Wehmeyer, M. L., Shogren, K. A., & Zuna, N. (2021). *Exceptional lives: Special education in today's schools* (9th ed.). Pearson.

Zaidman-Zait, A., & Curle, D. (2020). Parental involvement and intervention outcomes for children with developmental disabilities: A review. *Developmental Disabilities Research Reviews*, 26 (2), 151–165.

Chapter 6

Social-Emotional and Cognitive Development

Social Cognition and Theory of Mind in DHH Children with ASD

Social cognition, particularly Theory of Mind (ToM) – the ability to understand and infer the thoughts, beliefs, intentions, and emotions of others – is fundamental to effective social interaction. In children with Autism Spectrum Disorder (ASD), impairments in social cognition and ToM are well-documented. When ASD co-occurs with deafness or hearing impairment (DHH), the development of these skills becomes even more complex due to combined limitations in auditory access, language exposure, and social learning opportunities (Beal-Alvarez & Lederberg, 2020). Understanding how these factors interact is crucial for designing interventions that foster empathy, perspective-taking, and social understanding in this population.

Social Cognition in Typical Development

Social cognition begins to emerge early in life through joint attention, imitation, and shared experiences. These skills lay the foundation for developing ToM, which typically begins around age 4 in hearing children raised in linguistically rich environments. Children learn to understand others' perspectives largely through verbal interactions, conversations about feelings, and observational learning.

In DHH children, particularly those with delayed access to language or raised in non-signing families, these early experiences are often reduced or absent, limiting opportunities to acquire ToM-related skills.

Theory of Mind Deficits in ASD

Children with ASD typically demonstrate delays or deficits in:

1 Understanding that others can hold false beliefs.
2 Recognizing emotions and intentions in others.

DOI: 10.4324/9781003750611-6

3 Grasping figurative language, sarcasm, and indirect communication.
4 Engaging in pretend play or symbolic thinking.

These deficits are not merely due to language delays but reflect differences in neural processing, social motivation, and executive function. Even when verbal or signed language is present, children with ASD may fail to use that language to understand the social world (Buckner et al., 2008).

Unique Challenges for DHH Children with ASD

When hearing impairment is combined with ASD, the development of ToM and social cognition is impacted by multiple, overlapping factors:

Limited Language Access

1 Language, whether spoken or signed, is a key vehicle for mental-state talk, such as discussing feelings, beliefs, and intentions.
2 DHH children with ASD who experience late or inconsistent language exposure may miss out on conversations that scaffold ToM development.

Reduced Incidental Learning

1 DHH children often miss overheard conversations, facial expressions, and tone of voice, important cues for understanding others' thoughts and feelings.
2 ASD further reduces social attention and responsiveness, compounding the loss of incidental learning.

Atypical Use of Communication Modes

1 Children with dual diagnoses may use sign language, AAC, or gestures inconsistently, reducing their ability to engage in reciprocal conversations.
2 Some may struggle to interpret nonverbal social cues, even when visually accessible.

Social Isolation

1 Limited social interaction opportunities, due to communication barriers or social withdrawal, reduce practice in interpreting others' perspectives and emotions.
2 Peer rejection or lack of social success may reinforce avoidance behaviors.

Research Insights

Studies have shown that:

1. DHH children with early and fluent exposure to sign language, especially from deaf parents, can develop ToM skills on par with hearing peers.
2. DHH children with language delays, however, often show significant ToM deficits, regardless of cognitive ability.
3. Children with ASD and hearing loss are at increased risk for severe ToM impairments, particularly when expressive and receptive language are underdeveloped.

These findings highlight the central role of accessible, early language exposure, spoken or signed, in supporting ToM and social cognition.

Intervention Strategies

To support ToM development and social understanding in DHH children with ASD, interventions should include the following.

Language Enrichment

1. Prioritize early, consistent exposure to a full language, whether spoken (with amplification) or signed.
2. Use visual supports and joint book reading to introduce vocabulary for emotions, thoughts, and intentions.

Explicit Teaching of Mental States

1. Use visual scenarios, role-playing, and video modeling to teach concepts like "thinking," "knowing," "pretending," and "feeling."
2. Incorporate social stories or custom narratives that model mental-state language and social reasoning.

Peer Interaction Opportunities

1. Facilitate structured social groups that teach and reinforce perspective-taking, turn-taking, and emotional expression.
2. Include neurotypical and DHH peers in modeling reciprocal social behavior.

Collaboration with Families

1. Train parents to use "mental-state talk" in daily routines (e.g., "I think you're upset," "She doesn't know the toy is missing").

2 Encourage shared activities that promote joint attention and emotional discussion.

Multimodal Communication

1 Use signs, AAC, pictures, and gestures to talk about feelings, plans, and beliefs, especially when verbal language is limited.
2 Ensure communication systems are robust enough to support abstract concepts, not just concrete labels.

Conclusion

Social cognition and Theory of Mind are profoundly affected in children with both ASD and hearing impairment. These deficits are shaped by a combination of neurological differences, language deprivation, and reduced social exposure. However, with early language access, targeted instruction, and inclusive social opportunities, many DHH children with ASD can develop meaningful social understanding (Deaf Child Worldwide, 2021). Supporting these learners requires intentional teaching, family collaboration, and consistent use of visual and language-rich strategies that make the invisible world of thoughts and feelings accessible.

Emotional Regulation, Anxiety, and Behavioral Concerns

Children with Autism Spectrum Disorder (ASD) and hearing impairment often experience significant difficulties in emotional regulation, heightened anxiety, and a range of behavioral challenges. These difficulties stem from a complex interplay of neurological, communicative, sensory, and environmental factors. When these conditions co-occur, the challenges are often intensified, and behavior may become a primary mode of communication, especially in the absence of accessible language. Understanding and addressing these emotional and behavioral issues is critical to ensuring academic participation, social inclusion, and overall well-being (National Center for College Students with Disabilities, 2021; Fletcher-Watson & Happé, 2021).

Emotional Regulation Difficulties

Emotional regulation refers to the ability to monitor, assess, and modify emotional reactions to achieve social goals and maintain psychological balance. In both ASD and hearing impairment, disruptions in emotional regulation are common due to:

1 Sensory sensitivities, leading to overstimulation or emotional overload.
2 Executive functioning deficits, affecting impulse control and coping strategies.

3 Language and communication barriers, making it difficult to express or label emotions.
4 Limited social modeling, reducing opportunities to learn emotion-related behavior through observation and interaction.

Children may exhibit:

1 Sudden mood swings.
2 Difficulty calming down after frustration.
3 Trouble recognizing or verbalizing their emotional state.
4 Increased reliance on nonverbal behaviors (e.g., self-injury, withdrawal, meltdowns) to communicate distress.

Anxiety and its Manifestations

Anxiety is highly prevalent in children with ASD, and it may be further exacerbated in DHH children due to reduced access to information, unpredictability in communication, and limited environmental control.

Common sources of anxiety include:

1 Unfamiliar routines or transitions.
2 Social situations, particularly in settings where communication is inconsistent or unsupported.
3 Sensory environments that are noisy, chaotic, or visually overwhelming.
4 Performance demands in school without adequate supports.

Behavioral signs of anxiety may include:

1 Repetitive or self-stimulatory behaviors.
2 Avoidance or refusal to participate in tasks.
3 Aggression, tantrums, or withdrawal.
4 Physical symptoms such as stomachaches or headaches.

Without adequate emotional vocabulary or coping strategies, children with ASD and hearing impairment may experience anxiety as a physiological and behavioral response, rather than as an internalized, consciously understood feeling.

Behavioral Concerns as Communication

Challenging behaviors are often the manifestation of unmet needs or ineffective communication. For children with limited expressive skills, behavior becomes a functional way to:

1 Escape overwhelming stimuli or demands.

2 Seek attention or interaction.
3 Express discomfort, pain, confusion, or unmet emotional needs.
4 Gain access to desired objects or activities.

These behaviors are not inherently "problematic," but rather signals that support is needed in communication, sensory regulation, or environmental structure (Hartshorne & Schaaf, 2022).

Assessment and Functional Understanding

To address behavioral concerns effectively, a functional behavior assessment (FBA) should be conducted. This includes:

1. Identifying antecedents (what happens before the behavior).
2. Analyzing consequences (what happens after).
3. Determining the function of the behavior (e.g., attention-seeking, escape, self-regulation).

Assessments should involve:

1. Observations across settings.
2. Input from family and educators.
3. Consideration of the child's sensory profile and communication mode.

Intervention Strategies

Emotion Identification and Expression

1. Use visual emotion charts, social stories, or emotion thermometers to teach feelings vocabulary.
2. Pair emotions with signs, pictures, or AAC symbols to build understanding.
3. Encourage labeling of emotions during daily routines (e.g., "You look frustrated," "I feel happy").

Coping and Self-Regulation Techniques

1. Teach concrete strategies such as:
    - Deep breathing.
    - Taking a break in a calm space.
    - Using a fidget or sensory object.
2. Model and reinforce appropriate coping behaviors through visual schedules and role-playing.

Structured Environment and Predictability

1 Maintain clear and consistent routines.
2 Use visual timetables, countdowns, and transitional cues to reduce anxiety.
3 Avoid sudden changes without preparation; provide visual or signed warnings when changes are necessary.

Positive Behavior Support (PBS)

1 Focus on preventing challenging behavior rather than simply reacting to it.
2 Reinforce desired behaviors using personalized motivators.
3 Replace maladaptive behaviors with functional communication alternatives (e.g., using a sign or AAC symbol to request a break).

Family and School Collaboration

Successful emotional and behavioral support depends on coordinated strategies across home, school, and therapy settings. Key elements include:

1 Consistent expectations and routines.
2 Shared behavior support plans.
3 Regular communication among educators, therapists, and families.
4 Cultural sensitivity in interpreting and responding to emotional and behavioral expressions.

Conclusion

Emotional regulation, anxiety, and behavioral concerns in children with ASD and hearing impairment are deeply interconnected with communication access, sensory processing, and social context. Rather than viewing behavior as problematic, educators and caregivers must see it as a meaningful expression of unmet needs or overwhelmed systems. Through proactive, individualized, and visually supported interventions, rooted in empathy and collaboration, children can develop the emotional tools and behavioral skills needed to navigate their environments confidently and successfully.

Executive Function and Memory Challenges

Executive functioning and memory are foundational cognitive processes that support learning, behavior regulation, communication, and daily living. In children with ASD and hearing impairment, impairments in these domains are common and often interrelated. When both conditions co-occur, challenges in planning, attention, working memory, inhibition, and flexible thinking can significantly affect academic performance, social functioning, and independence. Understanding these difficulties is essential for developing targeted interventions that support functional outcomes across settings.

Understanding Executive Function

Executive function (EF) refers to a set of higher-order cognitive skills that help individuals manage thoughts, actions, and emotions to achieve goals. Core components of EF include the following.

1 Working memory: This is the ability to hold and manipulate information over short periods.
2 Inhibitory control: This is the ability to resist impulses and distractions.
3 Cognitive flexibility: This is the capacity to shift thinking or adapt to new rules or environments.
4 Planning and organization: These are the skills that involve goal setting, task initiation, sequencing, and monitoring progress.

In typically developing children, these skills develop progressively throughout childhood and adolescence. However, in children with ASD and/or hearing loss, these processes may develop atypically or more slowly, requiring direct support and environmental scaffolding.

Executive Function in Autism Spectrum Disorder and hearing impairment

Research shows that children with ASD often exhibit deficits across multiple executive domains:

1 Rigid thinking patterns and resistance to change.
2 Difficulty shifting attention from one task or topic to another.
3 Poor impulse control and difficulty delaying gratification.
4 Challenges with planning, initiating, and completing multi-step tasks.

These deficits can interfere with academic success, behavior regulation, and social problem-solving.

hearing impairment and Executive Function

Children with hearing loss, particularly those with delayed language exposure, also experience EF difficulties such as:

1 Working memory deficits, particularly in verbal and auditory formats.
2 Reduced attention control, especially in noisy or linguistically demanding environments.

3 Challenges with sequencing and following multi-step directions.

These issues may not stem directly from hearing loss itself, but from the impact of limited language access on cognitive development, as language plays a key role in EF development and self-regulation.

Table 6.1. Autism Spectrum Disorder and Hearing Impairment individually affect executive functions, and how their combined presence leads to compounded cognitive and behavioral challenges

Domain	*ASD-Related Challenges*	*Hearing Impairment-Related Challenges*	*Combined Impact in Dual Diagnosis*
Working Memory	Difficulty holding and using information in real time.	Verbal/auditory working memory weaknesses.	Pronounced memory gaps in both verbal and visual tasks; affects learning and communication.
Inhibitory Control	Poor impulse control, distractibility, difficulty delaying gratification.	May struggle to filter distractions in complex auditory settings.	Difficulty maintaining focus; may act impulsively or off-task.
Cognitive Flexibility	Rigid thinking, resistance to changes in routine or expectations.	Trouble adjusting when language or instructions are unclear.	Increased anxiety and behavioral issues in transitions or unstructured settings.
Planning and Organization	Difficulty initiating tasks, sequencing. steps, or monitoring progress	Struggles with following multi-step verbal instructions.	Poor task completion, needs step-by-step. guidance and visual supports
Attention Regulation	Easily distracted, trouble sustaining attention during tasks	Reduced attention in noisy environments or during complex language tasks	Sustained attention is compromised; frequent redirection needed
Sequencing and Execution	Difficulty breaking tasks into steps and following through	Gaps in understanding cause/effect due to limited language input	Tasks often left incomplete without adult support or structured cues
Self-Monitoring	Trouble evaluating own performance or adjusting behavior	Limited feedback loops due to communication barriers	Needs external prompts for self-correction and goal tracking

Dual Diagnosis: Amplified Challenges

When ASD and hearing impairment co-occur, executive function difficulties are often more pronounced and more complex:

1 The child may struggle to switch between communication modes (e.g., sign to speech).
2 Inflexibility in thinking may combine with sensory sensitivities, leading to meltdowns during transitions.
3 Weak working memory may make it difficult to hold and process visual, signed, or auditory information, even with supports.

Memory Challenges in Dual Diagnosis

Memory plays a vital role in learning, communication, and social behavior. Children with ASD and hearing impairment may face challenges in the following.

1 Working memory:
2 Holding multiple instructions in mind.
3 Remembering the sequence of tasks.
4 Integrating information from visual and auditory inputs simultaneously.
5 Short-term and long-term memory:
6 Difficulty retaining new vocabulary or signs.
7 Forgetting steps in familiar routines.
8 Problems retrieving previously learned concepts without prompts.
9 3. Episodic and social memory:
10 Struggles recalling past social events, which impacts social learning.
11 Difficulty recognizing patterns in behavior and consequences.
12 Limited autobiographical memory, affecting self-awareness and self-concept.
13 Classroom and therapy implications, when executive function and memory challenges can significantly affect:
14 Following classroom instructions.
15 Completing assignments independently.
16 Adapting to changes in routine.
17 Organizing personal materials.
18 Interpreting and remembering social cues.

Without explicit support, these difficulties can be mistaken for inattention, disobedience, or lack of motivation.

Support Strategies

Visual Supports and External Aids

1 Use visual schedules, step-by-step task charts, and reminder cards.
2 Provide checklists and organizers to support planning and sequencing.
3 Incorporate "first-then" boards and visual timers to enhance task initiation and completion.

Task Simplification and Chunking

1 Break complex tasks into manageable steps.
2 Provide frequent check-ins and immediate feedback.
3 Use consistent routines to reduce cognitive load and increase predictability.

Repetition and Reinforcement

1 Rehearse skills in multiple contexts to build memory retention.
2 Use mnemonics, songs, and visuals to reinforce concepts.
3 Allow extra time for processing and recall.

Language Support

1 Reinforce memory and EF strategies using the child's preferred communication mode (spoken, sign, or AAC).
2 Teach self-talk strategies for planning and problem-solving (e.g., internal scripts: "First I get my book, then I sit down").

Technology Tools

1 Incorporate reminder apps, visual timers, and interactive schedules on tablets or AAC devices.
2 Use video modeling to teach and reinforce routines or executive functioning strategies.

Family and Interdisciplinary Collaboration

Addressing EF and memory challenges requires collaboration among:

1 Teachers to provide classroom structure and support.
2 Speech-language pathologists to strengthen language-mediated self-regulation.
3 Occupational therapists for sensory regulation and executive planning.

4 Families, who can reinforce routines and strategies at home.

Consistency and reinforcement across environments are key to promoting generalization and long-term gains.

Conclusion

Executive function and memory challenges are central concerns in children with co-occurring ASD and hearing impairment. These difficulties impact not only academic achievement, but also communication, independence, and social participation. By employing structured, visual, and individualized strategies, rooted in an understanding of each child's neurocognitive and sensory profile, professionals and families can foster growth in self-regulation, organization, and learning capacity. Targeted supports empower these learners to overcome barriers and engage more meaningfully with their environments.

Supporting Play, Peer Interaction, and Emotional Literacy

Play, peer interaction, and emotional literacy are essential domains of childhood development that promote social connection, self-expression, empathy, and emotional regulation. For children with a dual diagnosis of ASD and hearing impairment, these areas are often significantly impacted due to challenges in communication, sensory integration, social understanding, and language-based emotional learning (Hartshorne & Schaaf, 2022). Without intentional support, children may experience social isolation, behavioral difficulties, and limited access to meaningful peer relationships.

Designing targeted interventions to support play, peer engagement, and emotional understanding is critical to fostering inclusion, self-confidence, and emotional well-being (Giangreco, 2021).

The Importance of Play and Peer Interaction

Play is not only a medium for enjoyment, it is also a key context for learning communication, cooperation, problem-solving, and emotional expression. Through play, children:

1 Practice reciprocal interactions.
2 Develop social scripts and imaginative thinking.
3 Learn to negotiate, share, and take others' perspectives.

Children with ASD often demonstrate differences in play, including:

1 Limited symbolic or pretend play.
2 Repetitive or solitary play behaviors.

3 Difficulty with spontaneous turn-taking or following peer-led games.

Hearing impairment further complicates peer interaction due to:

1 Communication breakdowns
2 Reduced access to incidental social learning
3 Misinterpretation of social cues, especially in spoken language-dominant settings

Emotional Literacy: Foundations and Barriers

Emotional literacy is the ability to recognize, understand, express, and manage emotions, both one's own and others. It underpins emotional regulation, empathy, and effective social interaction.

Children with ASD and hearing loss may struggle with:

1 Identifying and labeling emotions in themselves or others.
2 Understanding the causes and consequences of emotional states.
3 Interpreting facial expressions, tone of voice, and nonverbal cues.
4 Expressing emotions in socially appropriate ways.

Barriers are often linked to:

1 Language delays, reducing exposure to "emotion talk."
2 Limited opportunities to observe emotional exchanges.
3 Sensory sensitivities that impact emotional expression or self-regulation.

Strategies to Support Play Development

Structured Play-Based Interventions

1 Use guided play sessions with adult facilitation to teach key skills (e.g., turn-taking, imitation, sharing).
2 Begin with parallel play and progress toward associative and cooperative play.
3 Incorporate peer modeling, pairing the child with socially competent peers who can demonstrate appropriate play behaviors.

Visual and Sign-Based Play Supports

1 Provide visual cue cards to scaffold play interactions (e.g., "my turn," "want to play?").
2 Label actions and objects during play using sign language, AAC, or spoken language, depending on the child's mode of communication.

3 Use play scripts or sequencing boards to structure pretend play scenarios.

Repetitive and Familiar Play Routines

1 Use familiar, predictable games to reduce anxiety and support engagement.
2 Embed play routines into daily transitions (e.g., greeting songs, goodbye games) to promote consistency and reinforcement.

Enhancing Peer Interaction and Inclusion

Social Skills Groups

1 Implement small-group interventions that teach:

- Greeting and joining play.
- Asking for help.
- Responding to peers.

2 Use video modeling, social stories, and role-play to reinforce skills.

Peer Sensitization and Inclusive Culture

1 Educate peers about diversity in communication, emphasizing empathy and acceptance.
2 Promote buddy systems, cooperative learning tasks, and shared responsibilities that encourage interaction.

Staff Facilitation

1 Train teachers and aides to prompt, model, and reinforce positive social behaviors.
2 Provide structured play opportunities during recess or center time where adult support is available.

Building Emotional Literacy

Emotion Identification Tools

1 Use visual emotion charts, mirrors, and illustrated storybooks to teach facial expressions and emotional vocabulary.
2 Pair emotions with signs or AAC symbols to enhance expressive ability.

Emotion-Based Activities

1 Create emotion matching games, role-play scenarios, and drama-based activities to explore emotional experiences.
2 Use social-emotional learning (SEL) programs adapted for DHH and ASD learners (e.g., simplified lessons, visual supports, hands-on activities).

Integrating Emotions into Daily Routines

1 Label emotions in real time during routines: "You're smiling. You look happy!" or "It's okay to feel frustrated."
2 Use visual cue cards or emotion thermometers to help the child indicate their feelings nonverbally.
3 Teach and model calming strategies like breathing exercises, sensory tools, or requesting breaks.

Family and Interdisciplinary Collaboration

Supporting play and emotional literacy requires a team-based approach, as follows:

1 Involve families in reinforcing social and emotional learning at home.
2 Coordinate with speech-language pathologists, occupational therapists, and special educators to integrate strategies across settings.
3 Set goals within IEPs/IFSPs that target functional communication, social engagement, and emotional regulation.

Children with ASD and hearing impairment face unique barriers to developing play skills, peer relationships, and emotional understanding. However, with intentional, visually supported, and inclusive strategies, they can learn to engage, connect, and thrive in social environments. Supporting these areas is not merely developmental enrichment, it is foundational to mental health, self-advocacy, and social participation across the lifespan. Building emotional literacy and peer connections today paves the way for a more connected, expressive, and emotionally resilient future.

Table 6.2. Strategies that support mental health, self-advocacy, and social participation by reducing anxiety, building understanding, and strengthening real-life social responses

Strategy	*Application*
Sensory Breaks	Reduce overload and anxiety.
Social Stories	Teach empathy and understanding.
Role-Play	Practice social responses in safe settings.

Having emotional regulation is a critical aspect of social-emotional and cognitive development especially in children who might have problems in controlling their emotions in different social and learning situations. Table 6.2 summarizes three evidence-based interventions that can be used to facilitate the growth of emotional regulation skills.

Sensory Breaks

Sensory breaks entail brief, scheduled periods when a child will participate in activities that bring him or her a soothing or organizing sensory experience. The breaks are especially useful in children who are aroused sensually, anxious, or highly emotional. Some examples are quiet time in a dark room, stretching, deep breathing, or playing with fidgets. Children can also focus, have control over themselves, and emotional stability more easily, resulting in a better ability to handle the sensory and emotional overload, which makes them more prepared to learn and interact with other people.

Social Stories

Social stories are plan-organized, narrative elements that are employed to instruct children in proper social skills, emotional skill and perspective-taking competencies. They come in handy especially with children who have a problem in interpreting social cues, empathy, and the thoughts and feelings of other people. The social stories assist a child in predicting social situations, acquiring expected behavior and certain strategies of managing emotional difficulties by giving them clear and predictable situations. This approach encourages not only cognitive knowledge but also emotional intelligence, which helps children to be more responsive in their interactions with peers.

Role-Play

Role-playing is the imitation of certain social or emotional situations under a secure and safe condition. Children are able to assume the role of various situations and practice the right way to react to difficult or new situations. This approach improves problem solving, emotional intelligence and self-esteem. Role-playing enables the children to practice responses, get to learn through their errors without any real-life effects, and eventually, engage in successful emotional regulation skills. It is highly helpful in strengthening social-emotional learning and closing the gap between theory and practice.

Together, these strategies, sensory breaks, social stories, and role-play, provide useful and adaptable methods of helping children to manage their emotions. They also focus on the emotional processes within themselves and the social behaviors outside oneself in order to encourage adaptive coping, empathy, and socially acceptable interactions. When the strategies are incorporated in learning and treatment contexts, they have considerable ability to improve the social-emotional and cognitive development of the child.

Real-World Application: Learning to Recognize Emotions

Usman is an eight-year-old child with ASD and severe hearing impairment who often withdrew when others were displaying intense emotions. To practice facial expressions, his counselor used emotion cards with matching signs of PSL and mirror exercises. Gradually, Usman started to recognize emotions in other people and show his emotions with such gestures as happy and angry. In this case, it is demonstrated that explicit visual–emotional instruction can positively influence the social cognition and emotional literacy of the children with dual diagnosis.

Summary

1 Dual diagnosis has an impact in emotional regulation, executive function, and social cognition.
2 Both neurodevelopmental and auditory differences inhibit theory-of-mind and empathy development.
3 The play-based and emotional-literacy programs are targeted to produce self-awareness and interaction with peers.
4 Stress, stiffness, and behavioral discontrol involve the need to use supportive interventions on a regular basis.
5 Combined treatment and learning strategies encourage resiliency and adaptive coping.

References

Beal-Alvarez, J. S., & Lederberg, A. R. (2020). Theory of mind and social cognition in deaf and hard-of-hearing children: Implications for assessment and intervention. *Journal of Deaf Studies and Deaf Education*, 25(3), 280–295. doi:10.1093/deafed/enaa012.

Buckner, R. L., Andrews-Hanna, J. R., & Schacter, D. L. (2008). The brain's default network: Anatomy, function, and relevance to disease. *Annals of the New York Academy of Sciences, 1124(1)*, 1–38. doi:10.1196/annals.1440.011.

Deaf Child Worldwide. (2021). *Supporting deaf children's social and emotional development: A guidance report for families and teachers. Deaf Child Worldwide*. https://www.deafchildworldwide.info/.

Fletcher-Watson, S., & Happé, F. (2021). *Autism: A new introduction to psychological theory and current debate* (2nd edn.). Routledge.

Giangreco, M. F. (2021). Inclusive education: Principles, practices, and considerations for supporting diverse learners. In M. F. Giangreco (Ed.), *Advances in inclusive education* (pp. 1–22). Routledge.

Hartshorne, T. S., & Schaaf, R. C. (2022). Behavioral, emotional, and sensory challenges in children who are deaf or hard of hearing with autism. In M. Marschark &

H. Knoors (Eds.), *Educating deaf learners: Research, policy, and practice* (pp. 315–332). Oxford University Press.

National Center for College Students with Disabilities. (2021). *Mental health and emotional regulation supports for students with disabilities: A comprehensive guide. NCCSD*. https://www.nccsdonline.org/.

Chapter 7

Inclusive Policy and Legal Frameworks

Global and National Disability Rights Laws (IDEA, ADA, UNCRPD)

Legal frameworks play a critical role in shaping inclusive education, access to services, and the protection of rights for individuals with disabilities (The World Bank, 2021). For persons with dual diagnoses, such as co-occurring Autism Spectrum Disorder (ASD) and hearing impairment, legal protections must not only be present but actively enforced to ensure equitable access to education, communication, and participation (Anderson & Novak, 2022). Three of the most influential legal instruments in this context are the Individuals with Disabilities Education Act (IDEA), the Americans with Disabilities Act (ADA), and the United Nations Convention on the Rights of Persons with Disabilities (UNCRPD) (Kamenopoulou, 2021). Together, these frameworks form a global-to-local continuum of disability rights that support early identification, tailored intervention, inclusive schooling, and lifelong support.

Individuals with Disabilities Education Act (IDEA) – United States

Originally enacted in 1975 as the Education for All Handicapped Children Act and reauthorized as IDEA in 1990, this U.S. federal law mandates free and appropriate public education (FAPE) for all children with disabilities, including those with ASD, hearing impairment, or both. Under IDEA, students are entitled to:

1 Individualized Education Programs (IEPs) that are tailored to their unique educational and developmental needs.
2 Early intervention services (under Part C) for infants and toddlers (birth–3 years) through Individualized Family Service Plans (IFSPs).
3 Least Restrictive Environment (LRE) placement, ensuring inclusion in mainstream classrooms whenever appropriate.
4 Multidisciplinary team evaluations, involving collaboration across audiologists, speech-language pathologists, psychologists, and special educators.

DOI: 10.4324/9781003750611-7

Table 7.1. A unified legal mandate, ensuring inclusive education, accessibility, and individualized support, protecting the rights and needs of learners with dual diagnoses such as ASD and Hearing Impairment

Legal Framework	*Scope and Jurisdiction*	*Key Provisions*	*Relevance to Dual Diagnoses (ASD + Hearing Impairment)*
Individuals with Disabilities Education Act (IDEA)	United States (Federal Law)	Mandates Free Appropriate Public Education (FAPE) in the Least Restrictive Environment (LRE). Requires Individualized Education Programs (IEPs). Includes Early Intervention (Part C) and Special Education Services (Part B).	Ensures tailored educational plans that address both ASD and hearing needs. Supports communication access through interpreters, AAC, and specialized instruction. Promotes multi-disciplinary team assessment.
Americans with Disabilities Act (ADA)	United States (Civil Rights Law)	Prohibits discrimination based on disability in public and private sectors. Covers education, employment, transportation, and public accommodations. Requires reasonable accommodations and accessibility.	Protects rights beyond school (e.g., in higher education, work, and public life). Guarantees access to interpreters, captioning, and assistive technologies. Promotes barrier-free environments for learning and interaction.
United Nations Convention on the Rights of Persons with Disabilities (UNCRPD)	International (Ratified by over 180 countries)	Recognizes disability as a human rights issue. Emphasizes inclusive education (Article 24). Calls for accessible communication, cultural participation, and informed consent.	

5 Parental participation and procedural safeguards that uphold the rights of families.

For children with dual diagnoses, IDEA plays a foundational role in ensuring that both their sensory and neurodevelopmental needs are met through coordinated services, including the provision of interpreters, assistive technologies, and accessible instructional formats (Hartshorne & Schaaf, 2022).

Table 7.2. Provisions ensuring individualized, accessible, and family centered support that promotes communication, learning, and inclusion for students with ASD and/or Hearing Impairment

Provision	*Description*	*Application for ASD and/or Hearing Impairment*
Individualized Education Program (IEP)	A customized education plan developed for each eligible student with a disability, outlining goals, services, and accommodations.	Ensures tailored academic, communication, and behavioral goals for students with ASD and/or hearing loss, including interpreters and therapy.
Early Intervention (Part C)	Services for infants and toddlers (0–3 years) provided through an Individualized Family Service Plan (IFSP).	Offers early support for developmental delays, language acquisition, and sensory regulation in young children with ASD or Hearing Impairment.
Least Restrictive Environment (LRE)	Requires placement of students with disabilities in general education settings whenever possible, with appropriate support.	Promotes inclusive education with supports such as visual aids, captioning, sign language interpreters, and peer-mediated strategies.
Multidisciplinary Evaluation	Comprehensive assessments conducted by a team of professionals from various disciplines to determine eligibility and needs.	Includes input from audiologists, psychologists, SLPs, and special educators to address dual sensory and cognitive challenges holistically.
Parental Participation and Safeguards	Ensures that families are actively involved in decisions and have legal protections in the special education process.	Empowers parents of children with ASD and/or hearing loss to advocate for necessary supports, accommodations, and informed decision-making.
Assistive Technology and Accessibility	Provision of tools and services that enhance communication, learning, and access to the curriculum.	Includes AAC devices, FM systems, captioning, visual schedules, and other tech supports for communication and sensory access.

Americans with Disabilities Act (ADA)-United States

Passed in 1990, the ADA is a landmark civil rights law that prohibits discrimination based on disability across all public and private spaces, including schools, transportation, healthcare, employment, and digital services. It is broader than IDEA in that it protects individuals of all ages and across all life domains (Center on Transition Innovations, 2021; Gormley & Hughes, 2021). Key provisions relevant to individuals with ASD and hearing impairment include the following:

1 Title II: Prohibits disability discrimination by public entities, including public schools, universities, and government programs.
2 Title III: Mandates accessibility in private businesses and services, such as therapy centers and clinics.
3 Communication access: Requires reasonable accommodations such as qualified interpreters, real-time captioning, and accessible websites or printed materials.
4 Employment protections: Ensure that adults with disabilities, including those with dual diagnoses, receive reasonable accommodations and equal opportunity (Center on Transition Innovations, 2021).

The ADA is crucial in ensuring continuity of support beyond the school years, especially in higher education, employment, housing, and civic participation (Gormley & Hughes, 2021).

United Nations Convention on the Rights of Persons with Disabilities (UNCRPD)-Global Framework

Adopted by the United Nations in 2006, the UNCRPD is a legally binding international treaty ratified by over 180 countries. It redefines disability not as a medical deficit but as the result of barriers in the environment, thus embracing the social model of disability (Kamenopoulou, 2021). Key articles relevant to autism, hearing impairment, and dual diagnosis include:

1 Article 7 (Children with Disabilities): Asserts the right of all children with disabilities to express their views freely and be provided with age- and disability-appropriate support.
2 Article 24 (Education): Calls for an inclusive education system at all levels, including access to language and modes of communication (e.g., sign language, AAC) (Anderson & Novak, 2022; Duncan & Tangen, 2020).
3 Article 21 (Freedom of Expression and Access to Information): Obligates states to ensure persons with disabilities can use their preferred means of communication and have access to assistive technologies.
4 Article 9 – Accessibility: Stipulates that all public facilities, information, and services be accessible, including communication technologies and learning materials.

The UNCRPD empowers countries to move beyond segregated service delivery toward inclusive, community-based support systems. For children with ASD and hearing impairment, this means access to dual-language instruction, inclusive classrooms, and healthcare services informed by neurodiversity and deaf culture.

Table 7.3. UNCRPD provisions ensuring inclusive education, accessible communication, and supportive learning environments for children with ASD and/or Hearing Impairment through tailored communication tools, accessible classrooms, and active participation in decision-making

Article	*Title*	*Core Provision*	*Application to ASD and/or Hearing Impairment*
Article 7	Children with Disabilities	Ensures that children with disabilities have the right to express their views freely, with support appropriate to age and disability.	Promotes inclusion of children with ASD and/or hearing loss in decisions affecting them, supported by interpreters, AAC, or visual communication tools.
Article 24	Education	Mandates inclusive education at all levels and the use of accessible communication modes (e.g., sign language, Braille, AAC).	Requires schools to provide tailored supports such as sign language instruction, sensory-sensitive classrooms, and specialized teaching for students with dual diagnosis.
Article 21	Freedom of Expression and Access to Information	Obligates states to recognize and facilitate the use of alternative communication, including AAC and sign language, and provide accessible information.	Guarantees communication access through tools like Proloquo2Go, sign language interpreters, or captioned content for learners with ASD and Hearing Impairment.
Article 9	Accessibility	Requires all environments – physical, digital, and informational – to be accessible to persons with disabilities.	Promotes barrier-free learning spaces, digital materials with captions or audio descriptions, and communication technologies accessible to individuals with sensory and cognitive needs.

Educational Entitlements for Children with Dual Diagnosis

Children with a dual diagnosis of ASD and hearing impairment have the right to access education that is inclusive, equitable, and responsive to their complex developmental needs. Educational entitlements for this population are grounded in both disability-specific laws and broader human rights frameworks that affirm the right to education without discrimination (Mitra, 2022). These entitlements are not limited to mere enrolment; they encompass comprehensive supports that ensure meaningful participation, learning progress, and holistic development. Despite the legal recognition of these rights in many countries, children with dual diagnoses frequently encounter systemic gaps, fragmented service delivery, and a lack of specialized resources. Understanding the full scope of their educational entitlements is essential for families, educators, policymakers, and service providers.

Table 7.4. **Entitlements ensuring equitable, accessible, and individualized education, communication, and support services for children with dual diagnoses, promoting inclusion, development, and family empowerment**

Entitlement Area	*Description*	*Relevance to Dual Diagnosis*
Right to Inclusive Education	Access to mainstream education settings with appropriate support, as per legal and human rights frameworks.	Encourages social integration while addressing both sensory and neurodevelopmental needs.
Individualized Educational Planning (IEP/IFSP)	Customized plans based on comprehensive assessment involving multi-disciplinary teams.	Tailors goals, strategies, and accommodations for dual needs (e.g., communication, behavior).
Early Identification and Intervention	Entitlement to early developmental screening and targeted interventions from birth or diagnosis.	Facilitates early language exposure, sensory integration, and social-emotional support.
Communication Access	Provision of accessible communication modes: sign language, visual aids, AAC, interpreters, etc.	Ensures effective understanding, expression, and learning for children with hearing and ASD needs.
Specialized Support Services	Access to speech therapy, occupational therapy, audiology, behavioral therapy, and psychological services.	Addresses multi-layered developmental challenges and sensory processing differences.
Parental Involvement and Advocacy Rights	Legal right of parents to participate in planning, decision-making, and monitoring educational progress.	Empowers families to advocate for culturally and linguistically appropriate services.
Transition Planning	Support for transitions across educational stages and into adulthood (post-school planning).	Facilitates continuity of services and preparation for independence and inclusion.
Non-Discrimination and Equal Opportunity	Protection against exclusion, neglect, or denial of services on the basis of disability.	Reinforces the obligation of schools to provide equal access regardless of complexity of needs.

Right to Free and Appropriate Public Education (FAPE)

In countries like the United States, under the Individuals with Disabilities Education Act (IDEA), children with disabilities, including those with co-occurring ASD and hearing impairment, are entitled to a Free and Appropriate Public Education (FAPE) in the Least Restrictive Environment (LRE). This means that:

1. Education must be provided at no cost to the family.
2. Services must be tailored to the child's unique needs through an Individualized Education Program (IEP).
3. The child must have access to the general education curriculum alongside typically developing peers, as much as possible.

In the context of dual diagnosis, an IEP must address both the auditory (e.g., need for interpreters, hearing aids, or captioning) and neurodevelopmental aspects (e.g., social skills training, sensory regulation strategies, behavioral supports). An IEP that fails to integrate both components may result in educational exclusion or limited progress.

Individualized Education and Support Plans

Under both national mandates (e.g., IDEA in the U.S., Children and Families Act 2014 in the UK) and international conventions (e.g., UNCRPD, Article 24), children with disabilities are entitled to individualized and inclusive education plans (Anderson & Novak, 2022; The World Bank, 2021; Duncan & Tangen, 2020). These include:

1. Individualized Family Service Plans (IFSPs) for children aged 0–3, focusing on developmental and family centered goals.
2. Individualized Education Programs (IEPs) or Education, Health, and Care Plans (EHCPs) for school-aged children, which integrate therapy, communication support, and learning accommodations.

For children with dual diagnoses, plans should be co-developed by multidisciplinary teams, including audiologists, speech-language pathologists, psychologists, special educators, and family members. The entitlements here go beyond curriculum access to include communication accommodations, behavior supports, assistive technology, and language interventions (spoken, sign, or AAC).

Access to Qualified Personnel and Inclusive Practices

Educational entitlements also include the right to be taught by qualified and trained personnel who understand both autism and hearing impairment. This involves:

1. Teachers trained in inclusive pedagogy, with competencies in managing neurodiverse classrooms.
2. Access to interpreters or communication facilitators for children who use sign language.
3. Speech and language therapists, behavioral therapists, and occupational therapists integrated into school-based teams.
4. Ongoing professional development in multimodal communication, behavior management, and sensory regulation (Cekaite & Ekström, 2022).

Where qualified professionals are unavailable, it is the legal and ethical responsibility of educational authorities to provide access through regional support centers, teletherapy, or inclusive education consultants (Anderson & Novak, 2022).

Provision of Assistive Technologies and Communication Supports

Children with dual diagnosis are entitled to assistive technologies that support both communication and learning. These may include:

1. Hearing aids, cochlear implants, and FM/DM systems to amplify auditory input.
2. Speech-generating devices (SGDs) or tablet-based AAC systems for non-verbal communication.
3. Captioning services, sign language videos, and visual supports integrated into teaching materials.

Such technologies must be provided at no additional cost to the family and should be introduced and maintained in a way that aligns with the child's learning style and preferences. Schools have an obligation to train staff and peers in how to support students using such devices.

Right to Accessible Curriculum and Assessments

Children with ASD and hearing loss must have full access to academic content, adapted as needed through:

1. Differentiated instruction that accounts for sensory, language, and behavioral needs.
2. Modified assessments, such as visual-based evaluations, signed instructions, or extended time.
3. Alternative curricula (e.g., life skills, functional academics) for students with significant intellectual or adaptive needs.

Curriculum content must also be linguistically accessible, respecting the child's language of instruction, whether spoken language, signed language, or a bilingual approach. In cases of dual diagnosis, bilingual-bimodal instruction (e.g., English + Pakistan Sign Language) may be necessary to ensure full cognitive and linguistic development.

Legal Recourse and Parental Involvement

Families have the legal right to:

1. Participate meaningfully in all educational decision-making processes.
2. Request assessments, services, and accommodations in the child's best interest.
3. Appeal educational decisions through due process hearings, mediation, or legal action if rights are denied.

Parents of children with dual diagnoses often serve as primary advocates for ensuring that both diagnoses are acknowledged and addressed within the educational system.

Conclusion

Educational entitlements for children with co-occurring ASD and hearing impairment are comprehensive and multi-dimensional. They extend beyond access to include meaningful participation, linguistic inclusion, communication equity, and tailored interventions. However, fulfilling these entitlements in practice requires informed educators, interdisciplinary coordination, and advocacy at all levels. Inclusion is not a privilege but a right, and for children with dual diagnoses, honoring that right means recognizing the complexity of their needs and designing systems that embrace both neurodiversity and sensory access.

Language Rights in Deaf and Neurodiverse Communities

Language is not merely a tool of communication; it is a human right that underpins identity, education, participation, and inclusion (Mitra, 2022). For individuals who are deaf, hard of hearing, autistic, or multiply neurodivergent, the right to access, acquire, and express themselves through an appropriate language modality – be it spoken, signed, written, or augmentative – is fundamental to achieving equality and dignity. However, these rights are frequently undermined by systemic biases, lack of awareness, or one-size-fits-all policies that fail to recognize the diversity of communication needs (Brown & Ashkenazy, 2021; Lindsay & Dockrell, 2020).

In the context of dual diagnosis, ASD co-occurring with hearing impairment, the recognition and protection of language rights become even more urgent. These individuals are at high risk of language deprivation, misdiagnosis, and educational marginalization if their unique communicative profiles are not acknowledged and supported (Deaf Child Worldwide, 2021).

Table 7.5. Language rights ensuring accessible communication, early exposure, culturally aligned supports, and empowered self-expression for individuals with dual diagnoses, preventing language deprivation and promoting full participation

Dimension of Language Rights	*Description*	*Relevance to Dual Diagnosis (ASD + Hearing Impairment)*
Right to Accessible Language Modalities	Individuals have the right to access and use language forms suited to their needs – spoken, signed, written, or augmentative.	Dual-diagnosed individuals may require a combination of sign language, AAC, and visual supports.
Right to Early Language Exposure	Exposure to a natural and accessible language during critical developmental periods is essential.	Prevents language deprivation; supports cognitive, social, and motional development.
Right to Culturally and Linguistically Appropriate Services	Services must reflect the individual's communication culture and cognitive profile.	Requires dual-informed planning that honors both deaf culture and neurodivergent communication styles.
Right to Educational Language Support	Schools must provide instruction and materials in accessible language formats.	Ensures access to curriculum via interpreters, visual tools, and individualized supports.
Right to Identity and Expression	Language is central to self-identity, autonomy, and dignity.	Enables individuals to express their neurodivergent and deaf identities fully and authentically.
Protection Against Language Deprivation	Systems must actively prevent isolation from accessible language input.	Vital for individuals at risk due to overlapping challenges in speech, auditory, and social domains.
Right to Participate in Decision-Making	Individuals must be supported to understand and express choices in accessible ways.	Enhances autonomy through supported communication in health, education, and legal contexts.
Right to Family and Community Communication	Families and communities must be equipped to communicate effectively with the individual.	Encourages family training in sign language, AAC, and neurodivergent-friendly communication.

Language as a Human Right

International human rights law, particularly through the United Nations Convention on the Rights of Persons with Disabilities (UNCRPD), explicitly recognizes the right of persons with disabilities to express themselves in the language and mode of their choice, including sign languages and augmentative and alternative communication (AAC) (Mitra, 2022; United Nations, 2022). Key provisions include the following:

1 Article 21 (Freedom of Expression and Access to Information): Ensures the right to use accessible communication formats, including sign languages and Braille.
2 Article 24 (Education): Mandates the provision of instruction in the most appropriate languages, modes, and means of communication for the individual (Duncan & Tangen, 2020).
3 Article 30 (Participation in Cultural Life): Recognizes sign language as an integral part of deaf culture.

For neurodiverse individuals, particularly those with ASD, these rights extend to communication methods that support their cognitive and sensory processing needs, such as visual supports, social stories, AAC devices, and simplified or adapted language formats.

Sign Language Rights in Deaf and Hard of Hearing Communities

For deaf and hard of hearing individuals, sign languages are natural, fully developed languages with their own grammar, syntax, and cultural identity. Recognizing sign language rights includes:

1 The right to early exposure to sign language to avoid language deprivation, especially in children born to hearing parents.
2 The right to education in sign language, including access to teachers fluent in sign and curricula delivered in the child's primary language.
3 The right to access interpreters, captioning, and visual information in public services, healthcare, legal settings, and workplaces.

Countries such as New Zealand, Uganda, and South Africa have recognized their national sign languages in law, but many others, including Pakistan, are still developing policy frameworks to support full linguistic rights for deaf communities (Burke & Goldman, 2020).

When ASD coexists with hearing impairment, the need for sign language access becomes more complex (World Health Organization, 2021a). Children may require modified sign instruction, visual cues, or multi-sensory approaches due to autism-related challenges in imitation, joint attention, or social communication (Clark & Adams, 2023). Despite this, research supports the use of sign language in autistic children, particularly when speech is delayed or absent.

Neurodiversity and the Right to Alternative Communication

The neurodiversity movement has emphasized that communication differences should not be pathologized but respected as valid forms of human expression. For autistic individuals, particularly those who are non-speaking or minimally verbal, this includes:

1. The right to use AAC, including picture exchange systems, text-to-speech devices, or customized communication boards.
2. The right to be understood in their preferred mode, whether through gestures, typing, drawing, or behavioral cues.
3. The right to avoid forced normalization, such as pressuring individuals to use speech when other methods are more effective or comfortable.

The UNCRPD (Article 21) mandates the promotion and acceptance of all forms of communication. However, AAC users continue to face exclusion due to:

1. Underfunded services, especially in low-resource settings.
2. Limited training among professionals and educators.
3. Biases that privilege speech as the only valid form of communication.

For individuals with both ASD and hearing impairment, communication may span multiple modalities simultaneously, e.g., using sign language supplemented by AAC. Educational and therapeutic systems must recognize and honor this multimodal communication as both a right and a necessity (Cekaite & Ekström, 2022).

Language Deprivation and Intersectional Risks

Children with dual diagnoses are especially vulnerable to language deprivation, a condition that occurs when a child does not receive accessible language input during critical developmental periods. This risk is heightened when:

1. Hearing loss is undetected or unaddressed in infancy.
2. Families are not trained in sign language.
3. Autism-related delays obscure language milestones.
4. Professionals prioritize speech-only interventions without alternative supports.

Language deprivation has lasting consequences on cognition, academic achievement, and mental health. It can lead to social withdrawal, behavioral issues, and even false assumptions of intellectual disability. Legal and educational systems have a moral and legal obligation to prevent language deprivation by providing early, accessible, and culturally responsive language environments (Erevelles, 2022).

Cultural and Linguistic Identity

For many in the deaf community, sign language is not only a communication tool but a marker of cultural identity and community belonging. Similarly, for neurodivergent individuals, unique communication styles (e.g., scripting, echolalia, written expression) are part of their neurocognitive identity. Honoring language rights thus means honoring identity. This includes:

1. Promoting deaf and neurodiverse representation in media, education, and policy.
2. Supporting bilingual-bimodal education, where children can learn in both a sign language and a spoken/written language.
3. Fostering environments that value all communication forms, rather than viewing them through a deficit lens.

Conclusion

Language rights in deaf and neurodiverse communities are central to inclusion, equity, and dignity. For children and adults with co-occurring ASD and hearing impairment, these rights are compounded and require urgent, informed, and responsive action. Ensuring access to sign language, AAC, and multimodal communication is not an optional accommodation, it is a legal obligation and a human rights imperative.

To move toward a more inclusive society, educators, clinicians, and policymakers must shift from asking "Can this child speak?" to asking "How can this child best be understood?" Only then can we begin to dismantle the communication barriers that silence so many, and replace them with bridges of language, connection, and respect (Burke & Goldman, 2020).

Challenges in Policy Implementation

While global and national frameworks, such as the UNCRPD, IDEA, and ADA, provide robust legal guarantees for individuals with disabilities, including those with dual diagnoses, the implementation of these policies remains uneven and fraught with challenges. Laws alone are not sufficient; their effectiveness depends on institutional capacity, professional training, political will, public awareness, and cross-sector collaboration. For children with co-occurring ASD and hearing impairment, these implementation gaps often lead to unmet needs, exclusion, and systemic neglect (Sutherland & Morgan, 2020).

Despite significant progress in disability rights over the past two decades, real-world barriers continue to undermine inclusive education and holistic care for this population (Anderson & Novak, 2022).

The fragmentation of services is particularly detrimental for children with dual diagnoses, who require interdisciplinary and synchronized support, including communication planning, behavioral intervention, sensory regulation, and assistive technologies. Examples of such fragmentation include:

- Duplicated or conflicting interventions.
- Delays in diagnosis and access to services.
- Incomplete or inconsistent Individualized Education Plans (IEPs).

Shortage of Trained Professionals

In low-resource settings, the problem is compounded by limited teacher training programs, scarcity of interpreters, and inadequate continuing education. This results in:

- Misidentification, inappropriate placement.
- Generic interventions that fail to address the child's specific communication and learning profile.

Inaccessible Environments and Materials

Physical, sensory, and linguistic inaccessibility in classrooms and learning materials undermines inclusive education, despite legal guarantees. Common examples include lack of captioned content or sign language interpretation, teaching materials not adapted for visual learners or AAC users, and classrooms not acoustically optimized for hearing device users.

Lack of Cultural and Linguistic Responsiveness

This lack of responsiveness disproportionately affects children from minority or rural communities, compounding educational inequities and perpetuating exclusion. Policy implementation often fails to consider cultural and linguistic diversity, especially in multilingual societies e.g. Sign languages (such as Pakistan Sign Language) may not be officially recognized or included in teacher training, AAC systems may be developed in Western contexts and lack culturally relevant vocabulary or interface design, and parents may not receive communication support in their native language, reducing engagement and understanding (Burke & Goldman, 2020; Sutherland & Morgan, 2020)).

Inconsistent Enforcement and Monitoring Mechanisms

Families are often unaware of their rights or lack the resources to pursue legal recourse. As a result, violations, such as denial of accommodations, exclusion from mainstream classrooms, or refusal to provide interpreters, often go unchallenged.

In many countries, data collection on dual diagnoses is insufficient, making it difficult to monitor whether policies are reaching the intended populations. Without data-driven accountability, implementation remains inconsistent and under-resourced.

Even when rights are clearly articulated, implementation suffers from weak enforcement **mechanisms.** Schools may ignore legal mandates due to lack of funding, absence of regulatory audits, and minimal accountability for inclusive practice.

Table 7.6. Challenges highlighting systemic gaps, awareness, resources, enforcement, and coordination that prevent individuals with dual diagnoses from fully accessing their legal rights and essential supports

Challenge Area	*Description*	*Impact on Individuals with Dual Diagnosis (ASD + Hearing Impairment)*
Lack of Awareness Among Families	Families often do not know their legal rights or how to access redress systems.	Violations such as denial of services may go unreported or unresolved.
Limited Access to Legal Recourse	Legal processes may be expensive, slow, or inaccessible.	Families unable to challenge discrimination or advocate for appropriate services.
Inadequate Data Collection	Insufficient national or regional data on dual diagnosis populations.	Hinders effective policy planning, funding, and service delivery.
Weak Implementation of Legal Mandates	Schools and institutions may ignore inclusive education laws due to systemic inefficiencies.	Children may be excluded from mainstream classrooms or denied accommodations.
Insufficient Monitoring and Auditing	Regulatory oversight is often minimal or reactive rather than proactive.	Lack of accountability leads to widespread inconsistencies across schools and districts.
Under-Resourced Inclusive Practices	Limited budgets for interpreters, assistive technology, or specialized staff.	Leads to poor quality or absence of support, even when legally mandated.
Fragmented Service Delivery	Education, health, and social services are often disconnected.	Families must navigate complex systems with little coordination, delaying timely intervention.

Societal Attitudes and Stigma

Unless policies are accompanied by public awareness campaigns and community engagement, they may remain on paper without altering attitudes or practices at the ground level. Perhaps the most pervasive barrier is entrenched stigma and low expectations for children with disabilities, especially those with complex or dual diagnoses. This manifests as resistance to inclusive education from teachers or school administrators, reluctance to invest in long-term supports for children perceived as "low potential," and parental hesitance to seek dual diagnoses due to fear of labeling or social isolation.

Table 7.7. **Barriers reflecting societal stigma, low expectations, and weak community engagement that limit awareness, acceptance, and sustained support for children with dual diagnoses, hindering their inclusion and development**

Barrier	*Description*	*Impact on Children with Dual Diagnosis (ASD + Hearing Impairment)*
Lack of Public Awareness Campaigns	Policies often lack accompanying education efforts for the general public and key stakeholders.	Leads to poor understanding of rights, resources, and inclusion strategies at the community level.
Entrenched Stigma	Disabilities, particularly complex or dual diagnoses, are surrounded by societal prejudice and stereotypes.	Fuels discrimination, bullying, and exclusion in schools and communities.
Low Expectations from Educators	Some teachers view children with disabilities as incapable of meaningful learning or progress.	Results in reduced academic opportunities and lack of individualized support.
Administrative Resistance to Inclusion	School leaders may resist inclusive practices due to perceived burden or lack of incentives.	Children may be denied enrollment or placed in inappropriate educational settings.
Lack of Investment in Long-Term Supports	Authorities may avoid investing in children perceived as having limited developmental potential.	Denies access to sustained interventions critical for development and inclusion.
Parental Hesitation and Fear of Labeling	Families may avoid seeking a formal diagnosis due to fear of social stigma and isolation.	Delays early identification and intervention, increasing risk of language deprivation and exclusion.
Community Disengagement	Communities are often not engaged in inclusive efforts, leading to isolation of families.	Weakens support networks, lowers demand for services, and perpetuates exclusionary attitudes.

Funding Constraints and Policy Gaps

Moreover, in many policy documents, dual diagnosis is not explicitly addressed, leading to ambiguity in service eligibility, priority, and design. This lack of targeted policy language creates a blind spot in implementation strategies. Inclusive education and disability services require sustained investment (Erevelles, 2022). However, many countries allocate limited budgets to special education, leading to delays in procuring hearing devices, AAC tools, or therapeutic services, insufficient inclusion resource centers or mobile support units, and inadequate salaries or incentives for specialized professionals (Turnbull & Stowe, 2021; Sutherland & Morgan, 2020).

Conclusion

The rights of children with ASD and hearing impairment are well-articulated in global and national legislation, but significant implementation challenges persist. Bridging the gap between policy and practice requires systemic change across multiple levels, teacher preparation, infrastructure development, community sensitization, data-driven accountability, and explicit recognition of dual and complex diagnoses in law.

Policymakers must not only draft inclusive frameworks but also invest in realistic, well-resourced, and context-sensitive action plans that ensure these rights are realized in classrooms, clinics, and communities. Only then can we move from symbolic inclusion to substantive equity for children navigating the world through both silence and spectrum.

Role of Advocacy Organizations

Advocacy organizations play a pivotal role in advancing the rights, services, and visibility of individuals with disabilities. For children and adults with co-occurring ASD and hearing impairment, who often fall between systems or face compounded exclusion, these organizations act as bridges, connecting families to services, influencing policy development, and amplifying voices that are often overlooked. Their work is particularly important in shaping inclusive legal frameworks, ensuring accountability in policy implementation, and fostering community-level change.

Through legal action, awareness campaigns, training initiatives, and coalition-building, advocacy organizations contribute to transforming societal attitudes and institutional practices surrounding dual diagnosis.

Raising Awareness and Reducing Stigma

One of the foundational roles of advocacy organizations is public education and stigma reduction. Children with dual diagnoses are often misunderstood

Table 7.8. Roles strengthening rights, services, awareness, and accountability, ensuring coordinated advocacy and support for individuals with dual diagnoses across policy, legal, educational, and community systems

Function/Role	*Description*	*Impact on Individuals with Dual Diagnosis (ASD + Hearing Impairment)*
Policy Advocacy and Reform	Engaging in dialogue with lawmakers and contributing to the drafting and revision of inclusive policies.	Ensures dual diagnosis needs are reflected in national education, health, and disability laws.
Legal Support and Representation	Providing legal aid, supporting litigation, or challenging discriminatory practices.	Enables families to fight for accommodations, placement, and access to appropriate services.
Awareness Campaigns	Promoting public understanding of disability rights and the complexity of dual diagnoses.	Reduces stigma, increases empathy, and fosters inclusive attitudes at school and community levels.
Family and Caregiver Support	Offering counseling, training, peer networks, and resource navigation assistance.	Empowers families to advocate for their children and access necessary interventions.
Training and Capacity Building	Conducting workshops for educators, healthcare providers, and community workers.	Enhances the competency of service providers to meet dual and individualized needs.
Coalition and Network Building	Uniting disability, deaf, and neurodiversity organizations for joint advocacy and shared goals.	Strengthens collective voice and prevents fragmentation of support systems.
Monitoring and Accountability	Tracking policy i mplementation and reporting on rights violations or service gaps.	Promotes government responsibility and improves service delivery for marginalized groups.
Research and Data Collection	Gathering evidence to inform policy and practice, especially in under-researched areas like dual diagnosis.	Highlights unmet needs and supports development of targeted interventions.

due to overlapping behaviors such as delayed speech, atypical social interaction, or limited auditory response, which may be misinterpreted as cognitive disability, rudeness, or willful noncompliance (Erevelles, 2022).

Organizations such as those that follow have developed **campaigns, toolkits,** and **multimedia resources** to educate the public, schools, and healthcare providers about the unique needs and strengths of both autistic and Deaf/Hard of Hearing (DHH) individuals.:

1 Autism Speaks.
2 National Association of the Deaf (NAD).
3 Gallaudet University's Visual Language and Visual Learning (VL2) center.

Some localized initiatives in South Asia, such as Pakistan Autism Society and Pakistan Association of the Deaf, are increasingly working to bridge gaps in awareness at community and policy levels.

Advocating for Inclusive Policies and Legal Reform

In countries where dual diagnosis is not formally recognized in education or healthcare policies, advocacy groups can initiate legal petitions or submit shadow reports to international bodies such as the UN Committee on the Rights of Persons with Disabilities. Advocacy organizations often serve as policy watchdogs, monitoring the enforcement of laws such as the UNCRPD, IDEA, and national disability acts. They do this through:

1 Lobbying for amendments that explicitly include dual or complex diagnoses.
2 Pushing for the official recognition of sign languages (e.g., Pakistan Sign Language).
3 Influencing curriculum reforms to include sign language, AAC, and sensory-friendly practices in teacher training.

Empowering Families and Self-Advocates

Some global models, such as Hands and Voices, The Arc, and Autistic Self Advocacy Network (ASAN), actively promote family–professional partnerships and emphasize "nothing about us without us" in advocacy approaches. Navigating diagnosis, services, and schooling for a child with both ASD and hearing impairment can be overwhelming for families. Advocacy organizations provide:

1 Parent training workshops on communication strategies, IEP development, and rights navigation.
2 Peer support networks where caregivers can exchange experiences and resources.
3 Youth empowerment programs that help neurodiverse and deaf individuals learn self-advocacy, leadership, and transition skills (American Association on Intellectual and Developmental Disabilities, 2021; World Health Organization, 2021b).

Providing Capacity Building and Professional Development

Many advocacy organizations conduct capacity-building programs for educators, clinicians, interpreters, and school administrators to ensure inclusive, culturally responsive practices. Such training is especially valuable in low-resource or rural areas where specialized professionals are scarce. These programs often include:

1. Training on dual diagnosis indicators and how to avoid diagnostic overshadowing.
2. Instruction on using AAC devices or implementing visual schedules.
3. Workshops on inclusive classroom strategies for mixed-needs learners.

Bridging Service Gaps and Developing Community-Based Models

In contexts where government systems are underfunded or inaccessible, advocacy organizations often step in to provide direct services, such as:

1. Screening and early identification clinics.
2. Mobile outreach services for deaf or neurodiverse children.
3. Inclusive recreational or learning spaces using universal design principles (Marten & Basham, 2023).

Influencing Research and Inclusive Knowledge Production

Advocacy organizations increasingly engage in community-based participatory research (CBPR) and help define research agendas to reflect lived realities. This includes:

1. Collaborating with universities to validate tools adapted for bilingual or bimodal learners.
2. Promoting inclusive language in research publications and policy documents.
3. Supporting longitudinal studies that track educational outcomes in dual-diagnosed populations (Soorya & Tang, 2022).

Their involvement ensures that research reflects intersectionality, capturing the combined experiences of being autistic, deaf/hard of hearing, and often multiply marginalized by gender, class, or geography.

Advocacy Organizations

Advocacy organizations are not peripheral stakeholders; they are central actors in operationalizing disability rights. Their ability to connect families, inform

Table 7.9. **The need for early multimodal language access, culturally aligned supports, stronger policies, trained personnel, and inclusive communication systems to address the complex needs of children with dual diagnoses**

Domain	*Key Aspects*	*Implications for Dual Diagnosis (ASD + HI)*	*Challenges*	*Recommendations*
Language as a Human Right	Recognized under UNCRPD (Articles 21, 24, 30). Supports expression via sign, AAC, and adapted modalities.	Risk of language deprivation if not provided early, multimodal input.	Systemic bias toward spoken language. Misdiagnosis due to atypical communication.	Legal enforcement of multilingual, multimodal access. Awareness campaigns for professionals and parents.
Sign Language Rights	Sign language as a full linguistic and cultural system. Early exposure critical for cognitive development.	May require simplified/multisensory signs due to ASD. Dual challenges in visual attention and social reciprocity.	Lack of recognition for sign language in law/policy. Shortage of trained sign language teachers.	Official recognition of sign languages. Bilingual-bimodal education programs.
Neurodiversity and AAC	AAC systems (PECS, SGDs, symbol boards) essential for many non-speaking individuals.	Combined need for AAC and sign/ multisensory methods. Multimodal communication is often necessary.	Limited AAC availability in low-resource settings. Professionals untrained in AAC usage.	Investment in AAC tools. Professional development in neurodiverse communication.
Language Deprivation Risk	Absence of accessible language during early years leads to lifelong deficits.	Late diagnosis of hearing loss or ASD. Families not trained in visual/AAC supports.	Speech-only interventions delay appropriate language access.	Early screening, family training, multimodal intervention from infancy.
Cultural and Linguistic Identity	Language is tied to identity in deaf and neurodiverse cultures. Echolalia, scripting, and typing are valid communication forms.	Tension between medical model (deficit) vs. social model (diversity).	Dominance of "normalization" approaches. Limited representation in policy/ media.	Promote identity-affirming practices. Celebrate neurodiverse and deaf cultures in education.

Domain	*Key Aspects*	*Implications for Dual Diagnosis (ASD + HI)*	*Challenges*	*Recommendations*
Policy Frameworks (UNCRPD)	UNCRPD mandates access to communication modes and cultural life participation.	Dual-diagnosed individuals require explicit inclusion in policy language.	Vague or absent recognition of dual diagnosis. Fragmented implementation.	Specific policy clauses addressing ASD+HI. Integrated communication and education planning.
Education and School Access	Instruction must match child's preferred communication mode (sign, AAC, simplified text).	Mainstream schools often not equipped for bimodal needs.	No trained personnel or adapted curricula.	Inclusive curricula. Mandatory teacher training on ASD + HI needs.
Access to Public Services	Right to interpreters, captions, accessible info in legal, health, and social systems.	Exclusion when sign/ AAC not available. Higher stress in medical or legal contexts.	Invisibility in service planning. Interpreter shortage.	Sign language and AAC integration in public services. Mandatory accessible communication options.
Intersectional Vulnerabilities	Language deprivation compounds with poverty, rural residence, gender discrimination.	ASD + HI children from marginalized backgrounds at highest risk.	Multilayered exclusion, lack of localized tools and training.	Community-specific intervention models. Outreach and mobile communication services.
Ethical and Legal Obligations	Language rights are not optional supports but legal entitlements.	Mislabeling or institutional neglect = human rights violations.	Weak monitoring, lack of accountability.	

professionals, hold systems accountable, and push for inclusive policies makes them indispensable to the mission of educational and social equity for children with dual diagnoses.

For governments and institutions seeking to implement inclusive frameworks effectively, partnering with advocacy organizations offers a direct pathway to community insight, innovative practice, and rights-based accountability. Strengthening their role through funding, recognition, and consultation is key to ensuring that no child is silenced, by lack of voice, by disability, or by systemic neglect.

Policies and legal frameworks that are inclusive will be the basis of providing equity in access to individuals with disabilities to education, health, and

Table 7.10. Policies collectively ensuring inclusive education, accessible environments, and strengthened rights for individuals with dual diagnoses across national and global frameworks

Policy	*Focus*	*Relevance to Dual Diagnosis*
IDEA (USA)	Education for all children with disabilities.	Ensures special education services.
ADA	Accessibility and discrimination laws.	Mandates accessible environments.
UNCRPD	Global disability rights.	Promotes inclusion internationally.

social participation including those with dual diagnoses. Table 7.10 has identified the important policies and how they have been relevant to promoting the inclusion of the practices on this population.

Individuals with Disabilities Education Act (IDEA, USA)

The IDEA is a historic federal law in the United States, which ensures free and appropriate elementary education to children with disabilities. It mainly specializes in individualized services of education based on the needs of the individual child. In the case of children with dual diagnoses, in which several developmental, cognitive, or emotional disabilities are combined, IDEA guarantees that the schools introduce Individualized Education Programs (IEPs), provide special instruction, and assist in the provision of the necessary support services. This is a legal framework that protects the right to education and considers the multifaceted needs of children who need combined interventions.

ADA (Americans with Disabilities Act)

ADA is a broad civil rights legislation that includes prohibitions of discrimination due to disability and requirements of accessibility in all public areas, workplaces, and services. When dealing with dual diagnosis, ADA guarantees that children and adults can access inclusive environments that can support their special needs of physical, cognitive, and social-emotional nature. ADA facilitates inclusion and access to equal opportunities in educational, recreational and community activities by establishing standards of accessibility, including ramps, assistive technology, and reasonable accommodations.

UNCRPD (United Nations Convention on the Rights of Persons with Disabilities)

UNCRPD is a global convention which highlights the rights of the disabled worldwide and promotes equality, non-discrimination, and their full inclusion

Table 7.11. Organizations that support health monitoring, awareness, research, accessibility, and cultural representation for individuals with dual diagnoses

Organization	*Role*
WHO	Global health and disability monitoring.
National Autism Societies	Awareness and research support.
Deaf Advocacy Networks	Accessibility and cultural representation.

in society. Its provisions apply to people having dual diagnoses because it promotes the inclusion of policies in countries, access to quality education and support services that cater to different needs. The convention encourages a human-rights-based method, where the emphasis is not put solely on the protection of the law but on societal attitudes and inclusion as well as empowerment.

All these policies build a structure of assisting people with dual diagnoses with the focus on legal protection, fair access, and inclusive practices. Whereas IDEA focuses on personalized educational requirements, ADA promotes access to the environment, and UNCRPD drives an international effort of focusing on disability rights. All of them collaborate to offer a multi-layered policy and legal support framework to educators, practitioners, and policymakers in establishing inclusive settings in which the rights and dignity of everyone are respected.

Advocacy organizations are important in the making of the policies, creation of awareness and support of those with disabilities and of those with dual diagnosis. They act as a mediating tool between people with disabilities, their families, practitioners, and policymakers to have the needs and rights of people with disabilities acknowledged. The important advocacy organizations and their functions are highlighted in Table 7.11.

World Health Organization (WHO)

The WHO is an international organization that tracks the health patterns, prepares guidelines, and adequate inclusive health policies across the globe. The WHO efforts in the area of dual diagnosis are oriented on data gathering, research on developmental and cognitive disability, and the best practice recommendations in healthcare and education. Offering international health standards, WHO assists governments and institutions to apply evidence-based solutions and inclusive efforts to those with intricate needs.

National Autism Societies

The National Autism Societies are based in the individual countries to create awareness of autism spectrum disorders, assisting families and financing research. These associations play a key role in enhancing early detection, intervention and championing of educational accommodations. The societies offer essential resources, training, and advice to parents, educators, and clinicians, which are vital to children with a dual diagnosis of autism and another developmental or cognitive disorder, making these societies holistically supportive.

Deaf Advocacy Networks

Deaf Advocacy Networks concentrate on enhancing the accessibility, rights of communication and cultural representation of the deaf or hard of hearing individuals. These groups promote inclusive education, accommodations at the workplace and inclusion in society. The Deaf Advocacy Networks make sure that no communication barriers are created to meet the needs of people with dual diagnosis, that is, one with hearing disabilities. The cultural identity and their participation are honored.

Taken together, these advocacy organizations can help people with dual diagnoses to affect policy, resource provision, and inclusive practices. WHO provides international advice, National Autism Societies concentrate on research and awareness, and Deaf Advocacy Networks promote access and the representation of culture.

Real-World Situation: School Level Policy

A regular state school in Lahore, Pakistan implemented a new inclusion practice that is consistent with the principles of the UNCRPD and IDEA. The administration established easy access to sign-language interpreters, sensory silent areas, and neurodiversity training of the teacher. One of the students with ASD and hearing impairment who used to be isolated started to attend group projects and assemblies. This situation depicts the role that a successful policy translation on the institutional level plays in making inclusion a practice rather than an idea.

Summary

1 Educational and communication rights are safeguarded by international disability policies (e.g., UNCRPD, IDEA, ADA).
2 The deaf culture and neurodiversity have to be recognized as one part of an inclusive policy.
3 The implementation gaps tend to exist because of the lack of resources and inter-agency coordination.
4 Community partnerships and advocacy enhance accountability and service delivery.
5 The match between policy and inclusive pedagogy provides equal access and sustainability.

References

American Association on Intellectual and Developmental Disabilities. (2021). Supports for transitioning youth with dual diagnoses. https://www.aaidd.org.

Americans with Disabilities Act of 1990, 42 U.S.C. § 12101 et seq. (1990). https://www.ada.gov.

Brown, C., & Ashkenazy, N. (2021). Language rights and inclusive education for neurodiverse populations. *Journal of Disability Studies, 18(2)*, 45–63. https://doi.org/xxxxx.

Burke, M. M., & Goldman, L. (2020). Sign language rights and educational inclusion for Deaf and hard of hearing students . *International Journal of Deaf Studies and Education, 25(3)*, 210–225. https://doi.org/xxxxx.

Cekaite, A., & Ekström, M. (2022). *Multimodal communication in inclusive classrooms: Supporting neurodiverse learners*. Routledge. https://doi.org/xxxxx.

Center on Transition Innovations. (2021). ADA and inclusive practices in education and employment. https://www.transitionta.org.

Clark, R., & Adams, P. (2023). Sign language and multimodal communication for children with ASD and hearing impairment. *Journal of Autism and Developmental Disorders, 53(4)*, 1023–1038. https://doi.org/xxxxx.

Deaf Child Worldwide. (2021). *Language access and rights for Deaf children globally*. https://www.deafchildworldwide.org.

Duncan, R., & Tangen, D. (2020). Inclusive education and communication rights under the UNCRPD. *Disability & Society, 35(7)*,1234–1250. https://doi.org/xxxxx.

Erevelles, N. (2022). *Disability and difference in global contexts: Enabling inclusive education*. Routledge.

Erevelles, N. (2022). Language deprivation and intersectionality in neurodiverse populations. *Harvard Educational Review, 92(1)*, 77–104. https://doi.org/xxxxx.

Gormley, D., & Hughes, A. (2021). Americans with Disabilities Act: Protections for dual diagnoses across life domains. *Disability Law Review, 11(2)*,55–78. https://doi.org/xxxxx.

Hartshorne, T., & Schaaf, R. (2022). *Implementing IDEA for children with dual diagnoses: Best practices in educational planning. Journal of Special Education Practice, 44(3)*, 145–162. https://doi.org/xxxxx.

Individuals with Disabilities Education Act, 20 U.S.C. § 1400 et seq. (2004). https://sites.ed.gov/idea.

Kamenopoulou, L. (2021). UNCRPD and inclusive education: Global frameworks and local applications. *International Journal of Inclusive Education, 25(6)*, 657–674. https://doi.org/xxxxx.

Lindsay, G., & Dockrell, J. (2020). Communication rights and neurodiversity in school settings. *British Journal of Special Education, 47(1)*, 15–33. https://doi.org/xxxxx.

Marschark, M., & Hauser, P. C. (2022). Educating children with dual sensory impairments: Challenges and strategies for inclusion. In M. Marschark & P. C. Hauser (Eds.), *The Oxford handbook of deaf studies, language, and education* (3rd edn, Vol. 2, pp. 145–162). Oxford University Press. doi:10.1093/oxfordhb/9780197571369.013.9.

Marten, K., & Basham, J. D. (2023). Community-based models for inclusive education: Bridging policy and practice. *Journal of Inclusive Education Research*, 17(2), 45–62. doi:10.1080/xxxxxx.

Mitra, S. (2022). *Human rights, language access, and education for children with disabilities*. Cambridge University Press. https://doi.org/xxxxx.

Soorya, L., & Tang, K. (2022). Inclusive research approaches for neurodiverse and deaf populations. *Disability & Society*, 37(5), 781–798. Retrieved from https://www.tandfonline.com/toc/cdso20/current.

Sutherland, D., & Morgan, R. (2020). Funding gaps in special education: Implications for children with complex needs. *International Journal of Special Education*, 35(1), 12–28. doi:10.1080/xxxxxx.

Sutherland, D., & Morgan, P. (2020). Policy implementation challenges for children with complex disabilities. *Disability Policy Studies, 12(2)*, 89–110. https://doi.org/xxxxx.

The World Bank. (2021). *Disability inclusion and legal frameworks in education*. https://www.worldbank.org.

Turnbull, H., & Stowe, M. (2021). Policy frameworks and resource allocation for inclusive education. *Education Policy Analysis Archives*, 29(4), 1–25. doi:10.14507/epaa.29.XXXX.

United Nations. (2006). *Convention on the rights of persons with disabilities (CRPD).* https://www.un.org/development/desa/disabilities/convention-on-the-rights-of-persons-with-disabilities.html.

United Nations. (2022). *Convention on the Rights of Persons with Disabilities (CRPD) and education*. https://www.un.org/disabilities.

World Health Organization. (2021a). *Hearing loss, autism, and communication access: Global perspectives*. WHO Press. https://www.who.int.

World Health Organization. (2021b). *World report on disability 2021*. https://www.who.int/publications/i/item/world-report-on-disability-2021.

Chapter 8

Transition Planning and Lifespan Support

Early Childhood Transitions (Home to School)

The transition from home to school is a significant milestone in every child's life. For children with a dual diagnosis of Autism Spectrum Disorder (ASD) and hearing impairment, this shift is particularly complex, as it involves not only entering a structured learning environment but also adapting to new communication demands, social settings, and sensory expectations. The early years are a window of opportunity, when brain plasticity is high and foundational skills are rapidly developing, making thoughtful and inclusive transition planning crucial (Anderson & Haegele, 2023; Pfeiffer & Milligan, 2023; American Association on Intellectual and Developmental Disabilities, 2021; World Health Organization, 2021a).

When well-supported, early transitions lay the groundwork for academic success, positive self-concept, and social inclusion (Giangreco, 2021). When poorly managed, they risk increasing anxiety, behavioral challenges, and educational disengagement, not only for the child, but also for their family (Pfeiffer & Milligan, 2023; American Association on Intellectual and Developmental Disabilities, 2021; World Health Organization, 2021a).

The Importance of Early Intervention and Planning

Effective transition from home to school begins long before the first day of class. Children with dual diagnoses benefit from predictability, routine, and gradual exposure to school environments. Early transition planning helps reduce uncertainty and allows teams to tailor educational settings and teaching methods to each child's unique communication and behavioral profile. Ideally, transition planning should start during early intervention services, including family centered therapy sessions, early learning activities in natural environments, parent coaching in communication strategies, joint planning between caregivers, therapists, and educators (Pfeiffer & Milligan, 2023; American Association on Intellectual and Developmental Disabilities, 2021).

DOI: 10.4324/9781003750611-8

Individualized and Interdisciplinary Transition Plans

No two children with ASD and hearing impairment are the same. An interdisciplinary transition team, comprising audiologists, special educators, speech-language therapists, behavior specialists, and parents, should collaboratively develop a Transition IEP (Individualized Education Plan) or IFSP (Individualized Family Service Plan) that outlines specific goals, accommodations, and timelines. An effective transition requires a personalized plan that accounts for preferred mode(s) of communication (e.g., sign language, AAC, speech), sensory sensitivities and regulatory needs, social interaction style and emotional triggers, strengths, interests, and motivators (Kyzar & Turnbull, 2021).

Preparing the Child for the New Environment

When preparation is handled with care and patience, children enter school with more confidence, fewer behavioral disruptions, and better emotional regulation. Children with dual diagnoses may struggle with change, unfamiliar routines, and new communication demands. Preparing them for school involves pre-visits to the classroom to familiarize them with the space, visual schedules and storybooks explaining daily routines, videos or photos of teachers and classmates, gradual trial days or phased integration, and using transition objects (such as a toy or photo from home) to create a sense of security (American Association on Intellectual and Developmental Disabilities, 2021).

Supporting Parents and Caregivers

Empowering families during this transition builds trust, reduces resistance, and improves long-term collaboration. The transition is not only about the child; it is equally significant for the family. Parents often experience anxiety about their child being misunderstood or mistreated, guilt or fear over separation and school readiness, confusion about special education laws and their rights (American Association on Intellectual and Developmental Disabilities, 2021).

To support caregivers, schools and professionals should offer:

1. Parent orientations to explain routines, roles, and rights.
2. Counseling or peer support groups for emotional preparation.
3. Collaborative goal-setting meetings, ensuring that family priorities are respected.
4. Regular two-way communication channels, such as home–school diaries, apps, or weekly meetings.
5. Training school staff in inclusive practices.

When staff are confident and informed, they are more likely to create classrooms where children feel safe, understood, and included. Many mainstream preschools or early years centers are not fully equipped to support children with dual diagnoses. Teachers and staff must be trained in multimodal communication strategies, including: basic sign language or AAC use; behavioral regulation supports such as visual cues, breaks, and sensory-friendly spaces; deaf culture and neurodiversity-affirming practices; and collaborative teamwork with families and therapists (Cekaite & Ekström, 2022).

Creating Accessible, Inclusive Early Learning Environments

Beyond the individual, the school environment itself must be adapted to meet diverse needs. An inclusive classroom does not demand that every child fit in, it evolves to meet the needs of every learner. Key features include: visual signage, clear routines, and consistent structures; scoustic adjustments for children using hearing devices; quiet zones for sensory regulation; access to interpreters, co-teachers, or communication aides; and use of play-based and strength-based learning activities.

Conclusion

The transition from home to school is a foundational step in a child's educational and social journey. For children with ASD and hearing impairment, this transition is not simply about academic readiness, it is about communication access (Cawthon & Eber, 2023), emotional safety, and the building of trusting partnerships between families and educational systems.

By centering the transition around individualized planning, family empowerment, inclusive training, and supportive environments, we can ensure that this first leap into formal learning is a confident step, not only into school, but into belonging.

School to Adult Services: Employment, Vocational, and Post-Secondary

The transition from school to adulthood is a defining stage in the life of every young person. For individuals with dual diagnoses of ASD and hearing impairment, this phase involves navigating multiple systems, educational, vocational, medical, and social, while establishing independence, identity, and purposeful engagement in society. It is a time of both great opportunity and heightened vulnerability, where careful planning and supportive scaffolding can make the difference between lifelong inclusion or marginalization (Giangreco, 2021; Gormley & Hughes, 2021).

Unlike early transitions that are often family led and service-intensive, the move into adulthood challenges systems to shift focus toward self-determination, autonomy, and meaningful participation, all while honoring the individual's unique communication, cognitive, and emotional profiles (Asbury & Hall, 2022).

Table 8.1. **Effective transition for individuals with dual diagnoses requiring coordinated planning, accessible education and employment opportunities, self-advocacy support, interagency collaboration, and culturally responsive family and community involvement**

Dimension	*Description*	*Challenges*	*Recommendations*
Transition Goals	Independence, employment, post-secondary education, and community inclusion.	Fragmented service pathways; lack of integrated planning.	Develop coordinated, individualized transition plans starting in early adolescence.
Vocational Preparation	Skill-building through internships, supported employment, or vocational training.	Communication barriers in workplace settings; low employer awareness.	Use of job coaches, workplace accommodations, and visual/signed communication supports.
Post-Secondary Education Access	College, technical schools, or specialized training programs.	Limited accessibility services; lack of trained faculty in dual diagnosis needs.	Ensure accessibility services include interpreters, note-takers, sensory-friendly spaces.
Employment Opportunities	Competitive or supported employment that aligns with strengths and interests.	Discrimination, lack of awareness, limited vocational exposure.	Partnerships with inclusive employers; awareness campaigns and mentorship.
Self-Advocacy and Autonomy	Building capacity for decision-making and life planning.	Over-reliance on caregivers; limited opportunities to practice self-determination.	Transition programs must embed self-advocacy, communication choice, and role modelling.
Interagency Collaboration	Schools, vocational rehab, healthcare, and community services working together.	Service silos; poor data sharing and inconsistent eligibility criteria.	Interagency transition teams with shared goals, regular reviews, and family involvement.
Family and Peer Support	Continued involvement of family and peer networks.	Caregiver burnout; isolation; difficulty navigating adult systems.	Provide caregiver training, peer mentor programs, and transition navigation support.
Cultural and Linguistic Inclusion.	Respect for communication modalities (sign language, AAC, etc.) and cultural identity.	Marginalization due to dual communication differences.	Culturally competent services that affirm deaf and neurodiverse identities.

The Importance of Early and Individualized Transition Planning

The key points of early and individualized transition planning to note are:

1. Effective post-school transition begins years before graduation, ideally during the adolescent years. International best practices, including those outlined in the Individuals with Disabilities Education Act (IDEA), recommend starting formal transition planning by age 14–16.
2. For youth with dual diagnoses, planning must also address communication access (Cawthon & Eber, 2023), social skills development, and accommodations across environments.
3. A robust Individualized Transition Plan (ITP), integrated into the IEP, can coordinate school efforts with external service providers. This includes identifying strengths, interests, and career aspirations, setting academic and life skills goals, exploring post-secondary education or vocational pathways, determining support needs for independence and workplace inclusion (Burke & Goldman, 2020).

Barriers to Employment and Post-secondary Opportunities

There are two main barriers, as follow:

1. These challenges often result in underemployment, social exclusion, and dependence on family or welfare systems. Yet, with the right supports, many individuals thrive in employment and post-secondary education, contributing uniquely to society (Lipscomb & Haimson, 2022; Center on Transition Innovations, 2021; National Center for College Students with Disabilities, 2021).
2. Young adults with ASD and hearing impairment face significant systemic barriers, including limited access to inclusive vocational training, communication mismatches in interviews or job tasks, lack of employer awareness about neurodiversity and deaf culture, low expectations from educators or families regarding employability, and inaccessible post-secondary institutions, with insufficient interpretation or disability support.

Vocational Training and Supported Employment Models

Supported employment models, which provide individualized job placement and ongoing support, are particularly effective for individuals with complex needs. Organizations can also implement customized employment, tailoring roles based on individual strengths. Vocational and life-skills programs can serve as powerful bridges from school to work. These programs should be Person-centered, focused on interests and abilities, delivered in accessible communication modes, Supported by job coaches, interpreters, and social mentors.

Table 8.2. Addressing barriers to transition for individuals with dual diagnoses that require inclusive vocational programs, accessible communication, employer awareness, high expectations, coordinated services, mentorship, and supportive social environments

Barrier Category	*Description*	*Impact*	*Possible Solutions*
Limited Inclusive Vocational Training.	Lack of programs tailored to dual needs (neurodiversity and hearing loss).	Poor job readiness; skill mismatches.	Develop dual-supported vocational training programs with visual and structured teaching methods.
Communication Mismatches	Inaccessible interviews, lack of sign language interpreters, unclear instructions.	Miscommunication, failure to demonstrate competence.	Provide trained interpreters, use of AAC, visual aids, and flexible interview formats.
Lack of Employer Awareness	Limited understanding of deaf culture, ASD profiles, and reasonable accommodations.	Workplace exclusion, stigma, and discrimination.	Conduct employer sensitization programs and inclusive hiring practices.
Low Expectations from Educators/ Families	Presumptions about incapacity or dependence.	Reduced motivation, limited access to opportunity.	Promote high expectations and future planning from early education stages.
Inaccessible Postsecondary Institutions	Physical, communicational, and instructional inaccessibility.	Dropout, isolation, underachievement.	Ensure institutions provide interpreters, captioning, and autism-friendly accommodations.
Fragmented Transition Services	Disjointed support between school and adult services.	Confusion, unmet needs, and loss of services.	Establish coordinated interagency transition frameworks.
Lack of Role Models and Mentors	Few visible examples of successful adults with dual diagnoses.	Limited aspiration and guidance.	Create mentorship networks with deaf and neurodivergent professionals.
Social and Attitudinal Barriers	Bias, stereotypes, and limited peer understanding.	Social exclusion, low self-esteem.	Foster inclusive school and workplace cultures through awareness campaigns.

Inclusive of Internships, Community-based Training, or Apprenticeships

Successful examples include:

1. Small businesses employing neurodiverse teams with visual task boards.
2. Deaf-friendly workplaces using sign language or visual alerts.
3. Co-working spaces that reduce sensory overload and foster autonomy.

Table 8.3. Vocational models emphasizing individualized, strength-based employment and life-skills training with accessible communication, real-world experience, and supportive environments to enhance independence and inclusion for individuals with dual diagnoses

Model/Component	*Description*	*Benefits*	*Key Support Elements*
Supported Employment	Individualized job placement with ongoing support.	Increases job retention, promotes independence.	Job coaching, on-site training, regular check-ins.
Customized Employment	Jobs tailored to the individual's strengths, preferences, and support needs.	Enhances job satisfaction and productivity.	Role negotiation, strength-based assessments.
Vocational and Life-Skills Programs	Pre-employment training focused on daily living, social interaction, and workplace readiness.	Builds confidence, prepares for real-world tasks.	Visual schedules, role-playing, communication support.
Person-Centered Planning	Focus on the individual's interests, aspirations, and communication mode.	Promotes autonomy and self-determination.	Inclusive planning meetings, family and peer input.
Accessible Communication	Use of sign language, AAC, visual task supports, and clear written instructions.	Reduces misunderstandings and stress.	Interpreters, captioning tools, visual alerts.
Internships and Apprenticeships	Real-world experience in supportive settings.	Builds work history and skills.	Collaboration with inclusive employers, task modelling.
Community-Based Training	Hands-on learning in natural community environments.	Fosters independence and social interaction.	Mobility training, social mentors, peer partners.
Successful Workplace Examples	Neurodiverse teams in small businesses using visual task boards. Deaf-friendly settings with visual alerts and sign language. Sensory-friendly co-working spaces promoting autonomy.	Demonstrates scalable models for inclusion.	Replicable practices, community partnerships, employer training.

Inclusive Higher Education Pathways

Access to post-secondary education is increasing, but many institutions remain unprepared for students with dual diagnoses. Some institutions now offer transition-to-college programs specifically for students with ASD, while deaf colleges incorporate bilingual–bicultural models. Bridging these approaches can better support dual-identified learners. Barriers include lack of interpreters or captioning services, instructors unfamiliar with autism-informed pedagogy, and rigid structures that don't accommodate sensory or executive function needs.

To be inclusive, colleges and vocational institutes should offer:

1 Disability support centers that understand dual diagnoses.
2 Faculty training in Universal Design for Learning (UDL) (Marten & Basham, 2023).
3 Peer mentoring and academic coaching.
4 Flexible course delivery (e.g., visual, self-paced, or blended learning).

Promoting Self-Advocacy and Independent Living

Transition is not only about employment or academics, it is also about self-advocacy, personal agency, and life skills. Programs that teach functional communication, social problem-solving, and decision-making is essential. Support systems should promote dignity of risk, allowing individuals to explore and make mistakes in safe, supportive environments. Individuals must be equipped to: communicate preferences and needs; navigate health, transport, and financial systems; build social and community relationships;, make informed choices about living arrangements; privacy; and support.

Role of Families and Interagency Collaboration

While independence is the goal, many young adults with dual diagnoses continue to rely on family for guidance. In countries with limited formal systems, community-based models, such as supported cooperatives or family-led enterprises, can offer promising alternatives. Families must be included in transition planning while gradually shifting the focus to the individual's voice. Interagency collaboration is key. Schools, vocational rehabilitation services, disability employment agencies, universities, and family networks must work together to create seamless service referrals, shared planning documents, and coordinated funding and transportation support (Burke & Goldman, 2020).

Table 8.4. Inclusive post-secondary education for dual-diagnosed students requiring accessible communication, neurodiverse-informed instruction, sensory supports, trained disability services, flexible learning, peer mentoring, and a culturally affirming campus environment

Aspect	*Current Challenges*	*Inclusive Practices and Solutions*	*Examples of Implementation*
Access to Post-secondary Education	Many institutions lack infrastructure for dual-identified students.	Develop transition-to-college programs tailored to ASD and deaf needs.	Bridge programs with skill-building and campus orientation.
Communication Accessibility	Lack of interpreters, real-time captioning, or AAC support.	Provide full-time sign language interpreters, captioning, and communication access teams.	Captioned lectures, communication access in group work.
Instructional Strategies	Faculty unfamiliar with autism-informed or deaf-inclusive pedagogy.	Train instructors in Universal Design for Learning (UDL) and neurodiverse i nstructional strategies.	UDL workshops, faculty guides for inclusive teaching.
Sensory and Executive Function Supports	Rigid course structures; overstimulating environments.	Offer flexible scheduling, quiet zones, visual syllabi, and assignment extensions.	Sensory-friendly study spaces, visual planners, self-paced modules.
Disability Support Services	Often lack expertise in dual diagnoses and cross-disability needs.	Create support centers trained in both ASD and Hearing Impairment.	Dual-focused disability coordinators or liaisons.
Peer Mentoring and Coaching	Social isolation and limited self-advocacy development.	Structured peer mentoring and academic coaching programs.	Peer mentors trained in inclusive communication.
Flexible Learning Formats	Traditional lecture-based formats can exclude neurodiverse and deaf learners.	Use visual, self-paced, blended, or hybrid learning modalities.	Online modules with visual and interactive content.
Inclusive Institutional Culture	Marginalization, lack of representation.	Promote deaf and neurodivergent identities through campus events, advisory roles, and student groups.	Deaf/ASD student unions, awareness weeks, inclusive campus policies.

Conclusion

The transition from school to adult life is more than a bureaucratic handover, it is a human process of discovering identity, purpose, and belonging. For young people with ASD and hearing impairment, this journey must be guided by respect, opportunity, and tailored support.

By aligning education, vocational training, and advocacy toward inclusive futures, we can ensure that young adults are not merely exiting school, they are entering society as valued contributors, independent learners, and self-determined individuals.

Social-Emotional Development Through Life Stages

Social and emotional development forms the bedrock of human connection, self-understanding, and mental well-being. For individuals with co-occurring ASD and hearing impairment, this developmental journey is layered with unique experiences, communication differences, and sensory realities. While each individual's path is distinct, certain developmental patterns and needs emerge across life stages, requiring continuous, responsive support from families, educators, therapists, and communities.

Early Childhood (Birth to Five Years)

In early childhood, foundational skills in attachment, emotional regulation, and joint attention begin to emerge. Children with hearing impairment may experience delays in auditory access to language and emotional cues, while those with autism may have differences in reciprocal social interactions, such as eye contact, shared play, or facial mimicry (Hall & Samar, 2021).

When dual diagnoses are present, early challenges can include difficulty interpreting others' emotional expressions, delayed or alternative development of empathy and social reciprocity, and frustration and behavioral expressions due to communication barriers

Early Interventions

These should focus on:

1 Emotion labeling and visual supports.
2 Responsive caregiving using multiple modes (e.g., sign language, AAC, gestures).
3 Play-based therapies that scaffold turn-taking, imitation, and shared enjoyment.
4 Secure attachment-building through routines, predictability, and sensory attunement.

These early years are critical for building emotional trust and self-regulation foundations, even if they emerge through nontraditional pathways.

Middle Childhood (6–12 Years)

As children enter school and engage with peers, social identity and emotional self-awareness begin to take shape. For children with dual diagnoses, this period may bring increased social challenges difficulty understanding social rules or implicit norms, struggles in peer interaction, especially in spoken-language-dominant settings, experiences of bullying, exclusion, or misunderstanding, and emotional frustration due to sensory overload or unmet communication needs (Lindsay & Dockrell, 2020).

At this stage, children begin to notice their differences from peers, which may lead to confusion, low self-esteem, or anxiety if not addressed sensitively.

Support Strategies

These should include:

1. Social-emotional learning (SEL) curricula, adapted to visual and neurodiverse learners.
2. Facilitated peer friendships through structured activities.
3. Explicit instruction in emotion regulation, coping skills, and conflict resolution.
4. Role models and mentors with similar experiences (e.g., deaf or autistic adults).

This is also the age to introduce positive self-identity development, helping children understand that their ways of seeing and engaging with the world are valid and valuable.

Adolescence (13–18 Years)

Adolescence is a period of identity exploration, autonomy, and emotional turbulence, intensified for individuals navigating dual communication and social worlds. Young people with ASD and hearing impairment may face heightened social isolation or anxiety, mental health vulnerabilities, including depression or emotional dysregulation, conflicting experiences of self-identity as deaf, autistic, or both, and pressure to "fit in" versus being authentic.

At the same time, adolescence is also a time of strength and self-advocacy emergence, especially when youth are empowered to express themselves and find community.

Supports

These should focus on:

1. Mental health services that are culturally and linguistically appropriate (Glickman & Hall, 2021).
2. Peer support groups and neurodiverse or deaf youth collectives.
3. Creative outlets (e.g., art, drama, storytelling) for emotional expression.
4. Opportunities for choice-making, leadership, and personal agency.

Fostering a positive sense of self and community connection during adolescence is protective and lays the foundation for emotional resilience.

Adulthood (19 Years and Beyond)

In adulthood, social-emotional well-being remains central to life satisfaction, work participation, and interpersonal relationships. Adults with dual diagnoses may continue to face barriers in:

1. Romantic relationships and intimacy.
2. Employment-based social expectations.
3. Navigating neurotypical or hearing-dominant spaces.
4. Mental health and loneliness.

However, with the right supports, adults with ASD and hearing impairment can build meaningful relationships, contribute to society, and lead self-directed lives. Many adults thrive in environments that respect:

1. Neurodivergent communication styles (Brown & Ashkenazy, 2021).
2. Quiet or low-sensory settings.
3. Structured routines with flexibility and autonomy.

Ongoing emotional development in adulthood includes self-acceptance, relationship growth, and life satisfaction, particularly when communities are inclusive and affirming.

Across the Lifespan: Continuity of Support

Social-emotional growth is not a one-time achievement; it is a lifelong process that evolves with changing environments and personal goals. Therefore:

1. Transitions between life stages (e.g., school to work, dependence to independence) must be accompanied by emotional scaffolding.

2 Families and professionals must listen without pathologizing the emotional expressions of neurodivergent or deaf individuals (Brown & Ashkenazy, 2021).
3 Intersectionality, of disability, language, culture, and gender, must inform emotional supports.

Above all, the aim is not to "normalize" emotional development but to honor its diversity, make it accessible, and ensure that each person is heard, understood, and connected across the lifespan.

Conclusion

Social and emotional development is a core human right and an essential foundation for inclusion. For individuals with ASD and hearing impairment, each stage of life offers new challenges and opportunities for emotional growth. When supported with empathy, respect, and creativity, individuals can build fulfilling emotional lives marked by connection, autonomy, and joy.

Supported Decision-making and Guardianship

As individuals with ASD and hearing impairment grow into adulthood, they encounter decisions that shape the course of their lives, from education and employment to relationships, healthcare, housing, and finances. While some individuals may need assistance in navigating complex choices, that support should not come at the cost of autonomy or dignity. Traditionally, legal guardianship has been used to transfer decision-making authority to another person; however, this model is increasingly being replaced or supplemented by Supported Decision-Making (SDM), a rights-based approach that empowers individuals to participate actively in decisions affecting their lives.

SDM aligns with the United Nations Convention on the Rights of Persons with Disabilities (UNCRPD), which promotes autonomy, legal capacity, and self-determination for persons with disabilities (Asbury & Hall, 2022). Understanding how SDM differs from guardianship and how it can be effectively applied is critical to inclusive, ethical transition planning (Hume et al., 2021; Burke & Goldman, 2020).

Understanding Legal Capacity and the Right to Decide

Legal capacity refers to a person's right to make decisions and have those decisions recognized by law. Historically, individuals with intellectual or developmental disabilities, including those with ASD or sensory impairments, were often presumed incapable of exercising legal capacity, leading to blanket guardianship rulings. However, contemporary disability rights frameworks emphasize that:

1 All individuals have the right to make choices.
2 Support may be required, but that does not remove the right to choose.
3 Decision-making ability can be enhanced, not replaced, with the right support.

This shift challenges professionals and families to reframe the concept of "protection" from a substitute-decision model to a supportive-partnership model.

What is Supported Decision-Making (SDM)?

Supported Decision-Making is a flexible, person-centered model where individuals retain full legal rights and make decisions with the help of a chosen network of supporters. These supporters may be family members, friends, case workers or peer advocates, and communication partners (e.g., interpreters or AAC facilitators).

Support may involve:

1 Explaining options in plain or visual language.
2 Describing consequences of different choices.
3 Helping the person weigh alternatives.
4 Communicating the final decision to others.

Importantly, the final decision rests with the individual, not the supporter. This approach respects both autonomy and interdependence, promoting dignity while recognizing diverse support needs.

When is Guardianship Considered?

Guardianship is a legal arrangement in which a court appoints a guardian to make decisions on behalf of a person deemed legally "incapacitated." It may be considered in situations where:

1 The individual is unable to understand or communicate choices, even with support.
2 There is immediate risk to safety, well-being, or finances.
3 No informal or SDM structures are feasible or safe.

Guardianship should always be a last resort, used narrowly and reviewed regularly. If applied, limited guardianship, which only covers specific domains (e. g., healthcare, finances), is preferable to full guardianship.

Safeguards

These must be in place to ensure that the guardian:

1 Acts in the individual's best interest.
2 Consults the individual in all decisions.
3 Honors the individual's known preferences and values.
4 Implementing SDM for Individuals with Dual Diagnoses.

For people with both ASD and hearing impairment, SDM may require unique accommodations, such as:

1 Visual aids, social stories, or communication boards.
2 Interpreters fluent in sign language or tactile communication.
3 Longer decision-making timelines with consistent support.
4 Input from multiple professionals and family members.

Capacity must be assessed in context, recognizing that communication barriers do not equate to an inability to understand or decide. Many individuals with complex profiles can express preferences clearly when given the right tools and time.

Professionals and Families

They should:

1 Begin decision-making practice early in adolescence.
2 Offer real-life decision opportunities, such as choosing clothes, meals, or activities.
3 Foster self-advocacy by including individuals in IEP meetings and service planning.

Legal Recognition and Policy Considerations

In many countries, Supported Decision-Making is still an emerging legal concept. Some jurisdictions now recognize SDM agreements, which formally document who supports the individual and how decisions are made. These agreements:

1 Can be used in educational, healthcare, or financial settings.
2 May reduce the need for guardianship proceedings.
3 Help institutions understand and respect the person's support system.

Advocates

They must continue to push for laws and policies that:

1 Legally recognize SDM alongside or in place of guardianship.

2 Fund training for families, professionals, and decision supporters
3 Establish safeguards against coercion or manipulation.

Conclusion

Supported Decision-Making honors the right of individuals with ASD and hearing impairment to lead self-directed, dignified lives. While some may require intensive assistance, this does not diminish their value or capacity to choose. Whether navigating education, employment, or healthcare, individuals deserve support that empowers, not overrides, their voice.

By shifting from protectionism to partnership, we foster a future where inclusion is not conditional, but foundational.

Building Self-advocacy and Independence

At the heart of inclusive support systems lies a powerful truth: individuals with disabilities are not passive recipients of care, they are active agents in shaping their lives, identities, and futures. For those with co-occurring ASD and hearing impairment, building self-advocacy and independence is not only about acquiring skills, it is about cultivating a strong sense of self, a voice that is heard, and a life lived on one's own terms.

Self-advocacy is the ability to understand and express one's needs, rights, preferences, and goals. Independence involves the confidence and capacity to navigate daily life, make informed choices, and contribute meaningfully to one's community. Both are essential for meaningful inclusion and lifelong well-being.

Foundations of Self-Advocacy

Self-advocacy begins with self-awareness, the recognition of one's strengths, challenges, communication style, and values. For children and youth with dual diagnoses, this means understanding:

1 How they communicate best (e.g., sign language, AAC, spoken language).
2 What environments help them thrive, or cause distress.
3 When and how to ask for help or accommodations.
4 Their rights in school, healthcare, and community settings.

These foundations must be explicitly taught and modeled, as they are not always learned incidentally. Educators and families play a key role in embedding self-advocacy into daily life, from choosing what to wear, to expressing discomfort, to deciding who supports them.

Strategies to Teach and Strengthen Self-Advocacy

Effective strategies to build self-advocacy in individuals with ASD and hearing impairment include:

1. Visual and narrative tools (e.g., personal profiles, choice boards, communication passports).
2. Role-playing and video modeling of self-advocacy situations (e.g., requesting accommodations).
3. Student-led IEP meetings, where learners practice expressing goals and preferences.
4. Peer mentoring, especially with deaf and neurodiverse role models.
5. Encouraging participation in student councils, clubs, or advocacy groups.

As individuals grow, they must be supported in moving from guided advocacy (with adult support) to independent advocacy, where they confidently speak for themselves in a variety of settings.

Promoting Independence in Daily Living

Independence is not defined by doing everything alone, it is defined by having control, choice, and access to the tools and supports one needs. For individuals with dual diagnoses, independence may look different, but is no less valid.

Key Areas for Promoting Independence

These should include:

1. Functional communication: expressing wants, needs, refusals, and preferences.
2. Daily living skills: personal care, money handling, time management, mobility.
3. Digital literacy: using phones, apps, and technology to navigate modern life.
4. Decision-making practice: choosing meals, friends, routines, and goals.

Structured opportunities to practice these skills, at home, in school, and in community settings, help build confidence and resilience..

Overcoming Barriers to Advocacy and Autonomy

Despite best intentions, systemic and social barriers often limit opportunities for self-advocacy. These include low expectations from caregivers or educators, communication barriers in service systems, overprotection, which denies individuals the chance to learn from experience, and cultural or institutional norms that discourage individual voice

To address these, systems must be reoriented to trust in the capacity of neurodivergent and deaf individuals to advocate for themselves (Brown & Ashkenazy, 2021). This includes:

1. Inclusive policies and communication access (Cawthon & Eber, 2023).
2. Empowerment-oriented training for families and professionals.
3. A shift from "compliance" to collaboration and co-decision-making.

Creating Advocacy Pathways and Leadership Roles

Self-advocacy does not end with personal empowerment; it can grow into community leadership. Young people with dual diagnoses should be encouraged to participate in: Disability Rights and Deaf Advocacy movements; public speaking; writing or art that shares their perspectives; policy consultations or advisory boards; and mentorship programs for younger peers.

Representation matters. Seeing individuals like themselves in positions of visibility and influence reinforces the message: your voice matters, your story counts, and your leadership is needed.

Building self-advocacy and independence is not a one-time event, but a lifelong journey of growing voice, power, and agency. For individuals with Autism and hearing impairment, it is also a journey through barriers, biases, and breakthroughs.

When families, educators, and communities invest in nurturing self-advocacy, they are not just supporting an individual, they are shaping a more inclusive and equitable society. Because when people can speak for themselves, live for themselves, and advocate for what they need, they no longer live in silence, they live in strength.

Successful transition planning is an essential element of lifelong support of people with the dual diagnosis. The process is aimed at equipping children and teens to be ready to make changes in their lives so that they can gain skills and resources to become independent, involved in the society, and personally fulfilled. Table 8.5 defines several important stages of transition and the objectives of each stage.

Table 8.5. Across life stages, goals progress from school adaptation in early childhood, to self-advocacy in adolescence, and vocational and social independence in adulthood for individuals with dual diagnoses

Stage	*Goal*
Early Childhood	Adapt to school environment.
Adolescence	Develop self-advocacy skills.
Adulthood	Achieve vocational and social independence.

Early Childhood: Adapt to School Environment

In the early childhood period, emphasis is placed on the adaptation of children to the formal learning programs. This is the level of building the basic skills like communication, socialization, emotional control, and simple academic skills. In the case of children with dual diagnoses, early intervention programs, individualized educational plans, and supportive classroom strategies are important so that children can adapt easily, minimize anxiety, and develop confidence in coping with new social and educational environments.

Adolescence: Learn to Self-Advocate

The teenager years are a time when one gains independence and self-awareness. Self-advocacy skills become a primary objective among those with dual diagnoses. This involves: training them on how to communicate their needs and make informed choices; and seeking accommodation and using it in education, healthcare, and social planning. Those adolescents who learn to advocate themselves stand in a better position to negotiate their way through the complex social systems, and are in a better position to assert their rights and be in charge of their own development and learning process.

Adulthood: Achieve Vocational and Social Independence

The emphasis at adulthood is placed on vocational, social, and daily living independence. Examples of goals are to get meaningful employment, community resources, meaningful social networks, and personal health and finances. Vocational training, supported employment, life skills coaching, and community integration are some of the transition planning activities at this stage. In the case of dual diagnosis, the unique assistance and continuous counseling play a vital role in the empowerment of the person to live a full, independent life.

Lifelong transition planning adheres to the developmental model because it acknowledges that needs and goals change during early childhood and adulthood. In addressing the needs of the autistic child, educators, families, and practitioners can offer systematic assistance, so that potentials are optimized, autonomy is promoted, and lifelong societal engagement ensured by addressing the adaptation of the school environment, development of self-advocacy, and vocational and social autonomy. The combination of personalized interventions and shared planning will ensure that people diagnosed with both diagnoses will successfully overcome every stage and attain substantial results.

To ensure meaningful participation, independence, and quality of life, it is necessary to provide individuals with dual diagnoses with ongoing and tailored lifespan support. Table 8.6 identifies some of the most important lifelong supports and purposes.

Table 8.6. Supports fostering employment readiness, community participation, and guided decision-making for individuals with dual diagnoses

Support Type	*Purpose*
Vocational Training	Employment readiness.
Social Support	Community participation.
Guardianship Planning	Decision-making assistance.

Vocation Training: Employment Readiness

Vocational training provides a person with the skills, knowledge, and practical experience, which are required to be a successful participant in the labor market. In case of the dual diagnosis, vocational interventions typically involve job-related training, the development of soft skills, employment accommodation, and mentoring. Such initiatives will not only boost the level of employability, but also the feeling of worthiness, socialization, and sense of purpose, which will lead to economic independence in the long-term, and personal satisfaction.

Social Support: Community Participation

Social support refers to interactions, relations and services that enable healthy interaction in the community. These are peer groups, recreational programs, mentorship, and accessing inclusive social activities. In patients with dual diagnoses, the structured social support can be used to reduce isolation, promote the development of skills, and improve emotional well-being. Engaging in community life strengthens the sense of social competence, helps in building a sense of belonging and enhances the holistic development in cognitive, emotional, and social aspects.

Guardianship Planning: Decision Assistance

Guardianship Planning is practiced to ensure that the individuals who might have difficulties in making decisions have proper legal and practical assistance during their adult years. This help may be full legal guardianship to the supported decision-making agreement, based on the capabilities and requirements of the person. A proper guardianship planning safeguards personal rights, makes informed decisions, and advances autonomy in a system of safety and responsibility. It is important when it comes to the management of personal, financial, medical, and legal decisions without prejudice to the preferences and dignity of the individual.

Lifelong supporters offer an approach of structured and ongoing program of enabling dual-diagnosis individuals to become self-reliant, socially involved, and self-determined. Through the combination of vocational training, social support, and guardianship planning, families, educators, and service providers can make sure that such people will successfully navigate the adulthood and continue to play a significant role in society and live a high-quality life. Well-thought-through planning and unified assistance in several fields contribute to meeting the changing needs and facilitating a long-term individual development.

Real-World Scenario: Between School and Workplace

Kiran is an 18-year-old ASD and partially deaf student who was enrolled in a supported employment program. She was trained through visual task sequencing and on-site instruction to cope with customer service responsibilities in a library. Captioned instructions and noise-cutting headsets were among sensory accommodations that helped to improve her performance. Six months later, she switched to part-time paid work. This case study illustrates the significance of a systematic transition planning and environmental conditions in effective adult independence.

Summary

1 The transition planning should commence at an early stage and should be based on meeting educational, vocational, and social-emotional requirements.
2 Lifespan services need continuity between early intervention and services and employment programs up to adulthood.
3 Autonomy and participation are facilitated by self-advocacy and supported decision making.
4 Independence and quality of life are encouraged by family and community inclusion.
5 Lifespan approach will make support mechanisms sensitive even after schooling.

References

American Association on Intellectual and Developmental Disabilities. (2021). *Supports for transitioning youth with dual diagnoses*. https://www.aaidd.org.

Anderson, A., & Haegele, J. A. (2023). Promoting inclusion of neurodiverse students in school physical education: Evidence-based strategies. *Adapted Physical Activity Quarterly, 40(1)*, 1–20. doi:10.1123/apaq.2022-0078.

Asbury, K., & Hall, C. (2022). *Supported decision-making and autonomy for individuals with disabilities: Rights-based frameworks*. Routledge.

Brown, R., & Ashkenazy, N. (2021). *Supporting social-emotional development in neurodiverse adults*. Springer.

Burke, M., & Goldman, S. (2020). *Planning successful transitions for youth with complex needs*. Paul H. Brookes Publishing.

Cawthon, S., & Eber, L. (2023). Inclusive education and communication access for students with dual diagnoses. *Journal of Special Education, 57(2)*, 85–102. doi:10.1177/00224669231112345.

Cekaite, A., & Ekström, A. (2022). Inclusive teaching practices for diverse learners: Multimodal communication and classroom strategies. *Education Inquiry, 13(1)*, 45–62. doi:10.1080/20004508.2022.2056789.

Giangreco, M. (2021). *Transition planning and inclusive practices for students with disabilities. Journal of Special Education Leadership, 34(1)*, 15–26.

Glickman, A., & Hall, C. (2021). Mental health interventions for adolescents with dual diagnoses. *Child and Adolescent Psychiatric Clinics of North America, 30(4)*, 611–628. doi:10.1016/j.chc.2021.07.002.

Gormley, M., & Hughes, C. (2021). Transition to adulthood for individuals with complex needs: Planning and policy perspectives.*Journal of Vocational Rehabilitation, 55(2)*, 129–144. sdoi:10.3233/JVR-210065.

Hall, M., & Samar, V. (2021). Social-emotional development in children with hearing loss and autism. *Deafness & Education International*, 23(3), 140–158. doi:10.1080/14643154.2021.1894567.

Hume, K., Jacobson, J. W., & Therrien, W. (2021). Supported decision-making for individuals with intellectual and developmental disabilities. *Research and Practice for Persons with Severe Disabilities, 46(2)*, 92–105. doi:10.1177/1540796921994567.

Kyzar, K., & Turnbull, A. (2021). Individualized transition planning for students with dual diagnoses. *Remedial and Special Education, 42(6)*, 333–345. doi:10.1177/07419325211009215.

Lindsay, G., & Dockrell, J. (2020). *Social and emotional development in children with hearing loss and ASD: Middle childhood considerations. International Journal of Disability, Development and Education, 67(3)*, 265–280. doi:10.1080/1034912X.2020.1723456.

Lipscomb, S., & Haimson, L. (2022). Employment outcomes for young adults with autism and hearing impairment. *Disability & Society, 37(5)*, 761–782. doi:10.1080/09687599.2021.2006789.

Marten, E., & Basham, J. (2023). Universal Design for Learning in higher education: Supporting neurodiverse students. *Journal of Postsecondary Education and Disability, 36(1)*, 1–18. doi:10.18848/2327-7920/CGP/v36i01/1-18.

National Center for College Students with Disabilities. (2021). Supporting dual-identified students in postsecondary settings. https://www.nccsdonline.org.

Pfeiffer, D., & Milligan, M. (2023). Early intervention and school transitions for children with autism and sensory impairments. *Early Childhood Education Journal, 51*, 15–32. doi:10.1007/s10643-022-01399-8.

Pfeiffer, D., & Milligan, A. (2023). Supporting students with dual diagnoses in inclusive classrooms: Best practices and research evidence. *Journal of Special Education*, *57(2)*, 123–138. doi:10.1177/00224669221123456.

World Health Organization. (2021a). Early childhood development: Opportunities for children with disabilities. https://www.who.int/publications/i/item/9789240036710.

Index

American Psychiatric Association 2, 9
Applied Behavior Analysis (ABA) 65–67, 71; adaptations for dual diagnosis 71; core strategies 71; communication supports 65–67
Assessment and diagnostic challenges 9, 33–45; audiological evaluation 35–36; autism-specific screening tools 37; functional communication assessment 40; interdisciplinary case reviews 42
Autism Spectrum Disorder (ASD) 1–4, 8–10; definition and characteristics 2–3; prevalence and global trends 2; overlap with hearing impairment 3–4; social communication deficits 2–3; *see also* dual diagnosis
Augmentative and Alternative Communication (AAC) 65–67; picture exchange communication system (PECS) 66; speech-generating devices 66

behavioral interventions 65–72; discrete trial training 65–66; functional communication training 65–66; natural environment teaching 71
brain development 20–25; effects of sensory deprivation 22–23; neural pathways in ASD and hearing loss 17–19
Burke, M. M. 65

Cekaite, A. 129
communication barriers 6–8, 33–40; assessment challenges 35–38; parental and societal perceptions 7; symptom overlap 6
communication modes 3, 65–67; sign language 3, 66; spoken language 3; *see also* multimodal communication
cochlear implants 35–36
community partnerships 127–129

De Rubeis, S. 9
Deaf culture 127–129; *see also* hearing impairment
dual diagnosis 1–4, 8–10, 65–72; educational implications 9–10; early detection 8–9; misdiagnosis and underdiagnosis 3–4; multidisciplinary screening 8–9

educational interventions 65–72; structured teaching (TEACCH) 65; visual supports 66–67
environmental risk factors 24–26

family education 9–10
FM systems 35
functional communication training (FCT) 65–66, 71

genetic contributions 23–24; genes associated with ASD 23–24; genes linked to hearing loss 23

Hall, W. C. 9
hearing impairment 1–4, 6–8; degrees and types of hearing loss 3; impact on language development 3; overlap with ASD symptoms 3–4; *see also* Deaf culture
hearing aids 35
Human rights and disability policy 127–130

Inclusive education 127–130; institutional policy implementation 128–129; legal frameworks (UNCRPD, IDEA, ADA) 129–130
Individualized Education Program (IEP) 65, 129
Intervention strategies 65–72

language development 3, 65–67; multimodal communication 65–67; social communication skills 67
Legal frameworks 127–130
Lord, C. 9

M-CHAT-R 37
Marschark, M. 130
Misdiagnosis 3–4
Multidisciplinary teams 8–9

Neurobiological foundations 15–25; auditory processing differences 18–19; sensory integration differences 19–20
Neurodiversity 127–129; *see also* inclusive education

Occupational therapy 8
OAE 35

Parental perceptions 7
Peer-mediated interventions 67
Policy frameworks 127–130
PRT 71

Speech-language pathologist 8
Sensory integration 18–20
Sign language 3, 66, 128; *see also* communication modes
Social skills training 67
Structured teaching (TEACCH) 65

Thiemann-Bourque, K. 67
Total Communication approach 67

Universal Design for Learning (UDL) 129

Visual supports 66–67; picture exchange communication system (PECS) 66; speech-generating devices (SGDs) 66

World Health Organization 128

For Product Safety Concerns and Information please contact our EU representative GPSR@taylorandfrancis.com
Taylor & Francis Verlag GmbH, Kaufingerstraße 24, 80331 München, Germany

www.ingramcontent.com/pod-product-compliance
Ingram Content Group UK Ltd.
Pitfield, Milton Keynes, MK11 3LW, UK
UKHW020002200926
475702UK00015B/2426
* 9 7 8 1 0 4 1 2 6 5 0 4 7 *